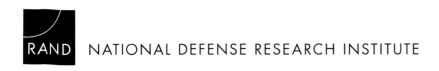 NATIONAL DEFENSE RESEARCH INSTITUTE

Understanding Treatment of Mild Traumatic Brain Injury in the Military Health System

Carrie M. Farmer, Heather Krull, Thomas W. Concannon, Molly Simmons, Francesca Pillemer, Teague Ruder, Andrew M. Parker, Maulik P. Purohit, Liisa Hiatt, Benjamin Batorsky, Kimberly A. Hepner

Prepared for the Defense and Veterans Brain Injury Center, Defense Centers of Excellence for Psychological Health and Traumatic Brain Injury

For more information on this publication, visit www.rand.org/t/rr844

Library of Congress Cataloging-in-Publication Data
ISBN: 978-0-8330-9276-2

Published by the RAND Corporation, Santa Monica, Calif.
© Copyright 2016 RAND Corporation
RAND® is a registered trademark.

Support RAND
Make a tax-deductible charitable contribution at
www.rand.org/giving/contribute

www.rand.org

Preface

Traumatic brain injury (TBI) has become a signature injury of modern warfare. For example, and although estimates vary, during operations in Iraq and Afghanistan, approximately 8–20 percent of service members may have experienced a TBI, with the majority (84 percent) being diagnosed as mild in severity. Many service members who have experienced a mild TBI (mTBI), also known as a concussion, receive care through the Military Health System (MHS). However, there have been no publicized, large-scale studies of the frequency and nature of post-injury health care use by service members diagnosed with an mTBI. To address this gap, the U.S. Department of Defense (DoD) asked the RAND Corporation to survey the current landscape of mTBI treatment across the MHS. Using the available data, the RAND study focused specifically on nondeployed active-duty service members. The goal of this research is to provide timely information to DoD that can be used to help assess and improve care for service members with an mTBI.

This report is the first of its kind to describe the characteristics of nondeployed active-duty service members who have received an mTBI diagnosis, their co-occurring symptoms and conditions, the locations where they received care, the types of treatment and medications they received, and the duration and patterns of their care. The analysis draws on individual-level health care utilization data managed and maintained by the Defense Health Agency, along with administrative data on service member characteristics, to identify and characterize nondeployed active-component service members who received treatment for mTBI in calendar year 2012 and the treatment they received through the MHS. The research team began by selecting a case definition for mTBI based on codes in the International Classification of Diseases, Ninth Revision (ICD-9), Clinical Modification. The team then used the case definition to identify all nondeployed active-duty service members who received a new diagnosis of mTBI in 2012 and examined six months of health care following the diagnosis. This report describes the findings from this analysis and provides recommendations for the MHS.

This report was prepared specifically for health policy officials, MHS personnel, and TBI program managers within DoD; however, the results should also be of interest to health policy officials in the U.S. Department of Veterans Affairs and the U.S. Department of Health and Human Services, as well as clinical and health services researchers examining the epidemiology and treatment of mTBI.

This research was sponsored by the Defense and Veterans Brain Injury Center in the Defense Centers of Excellence for Psychological Health and Traumatic Brain Injury and conducted within the Forces and Resources Policy Center of the RAND National Defense Research Institute, a federally funded research and development center sponsored by the Office of the Secretary of Defense, the Joint Staff, the Unified Combatant Commands, the Navy, the Marine Corps, the defense agencies, and the defense Intelligence Community.

For more information on the RAND Forces and Resources Policy Center, see www.rand. org/nsrd/ndri/centers/frp or contact the director (contact information is provided on the web page).

Contents

Figures

Tables

Summary

Of the approximately 2.5 million service members who have deployed to Iraq and Afghanistan in support of Operations Iraqi Freedom and Enduring Freedom, more than 50,000 were wounded in action, and between 30 and 50 percent of these injuries were the result of improvised explosive devices (IEDs; U.S. Department of Defense [DoD], 2014; Wilson, 2006). Traumatic brain injury (TBI) is a frequent consequence of IED incidents, so much so that it is considered the signature injury of modern warfare (Altmire, 2007; Clark, 2006).

Deployment-related injuries are not the only driver of TBIs, however. Such injuries may also result from training accidents, accidental falls, sports, and motor vehicle accidents. In fact, non–deployment-related TBIs accounted for 85 percent of all TBIs reported to DoD between 2001 and 2011 (Office of the Surgeon General, 2013).

Estimates vary, but studies suggest that 8–20 percent of service members may have experienced a TBI (Hoge, McGurk, et al., 2008; Schell and Marshall, 2008). Among those diagnosed with TBI, the majority of cases (84 percent) were considered mild in severity (Defense and Veterans Brain Injury Center [DVBIC], 2014a). Many service members who have experienced a mild TBI (mTBI), also known as a concussion, receive care through the Military Health System (MHS), but the frequency and nature of their post-injury health care has not been described in a large cohort. To address this gap, DoD asked the RAND Corporation to survey the current landscape of mTBI treatment across the MHS. The goal of this research is to provide timely information to DoD that can be used to help assess and improve care for service members with mTBI.

Mild cases of TBI can be challenging to identify and treat due to variations in symptom presentation and other factors. To deliver the most efficient and effective treatment for service members with mTBI, it is important to first understand how many and which service members receive an mTBI diagnosis, where they receive care, the types of treatment they receive, and the duration of their care. The ultimate goal of improving the care delivered to this population (and subsequent clinical outcomes) depends on a solid evidence base. This report provides a first step in establishing that base by describing the service member population diagnosed with an mTBI, their clinical characteristics, and the care they receive.

Because of the difficulty in accurately diagnosing mTBI and variability in screening procedures, there have been calls for clear and consistent definitions of study populations and standard guidelines for diagnosis (see, e.g., Helmick et al., 2012; Hoge, McGurk, et al., 2008). The research community has also highlighted the need to account for conditions often present with mTBI, such as post-traumatic stress disorder (PTSD) and depression (Carlson et al., 2011; Kristman et al., 2014). This report—the first comprehensive analysis of the types and patterns of care delivered by the MHS to service members following an mTBI diagnosis—aims to fill some of these gaps.

The findings presented here lay the groundwork for future research to assess and improve the quality of care by characterizing the population of service members who have received care for mTBI through the MHS, as well as the care that they have received, using health care utilization data. We began by evaluating multiple methods of identifying service members with mTBI using diagnostic codes from the International Classification of Diseases, Ninth Revision (ICD-9), Clinical Modification. Then, we drew on individual health care utilization records to characterize service members who received a diagnosis of mTBI and assessed the care they received, including the types of care, the settings in which the care was provided, and the types of providers who delivered the care. Finally, we explored patterns of care, describing health care received up to six months after an mTBI diagnosis, including the duration and patterns of utilization. In addition, we explored care provided to service members who received "persistent care," defined as care received beyond three months following an injury.

The results of this study are intended to support the MHS in its effort to deliver care more effectively and efficiently to service members diagnosed with an mTBI. However, they should also prove valuable to other health systems and health care professionals and officials involved with treating or setting policies regarding the treatment of service members and civilians with mTBI.

Identifying Service Members Treated for mTBI

For patients with a moderate or severe TBI, long-term outcomes can vary from full recovery to complete dependence on care providers. Measurable deficits in cognitive and physical functioning may still be present a year after the injury (Andelic et al., 2010; Novack et al., 2000). In contrast, symptoms associated with mTBI tend to resolve quickly for the majority of patients. Previous studies suggest that the majority of symptoms tend to resolve within the first month after an mTBI incident (Lundin et al., 2006; McCrea, Guskiewicz, et al., 2003), and, according to data on civilian patients, 85–90 percent with mild TBI recover within three months (U.S. Department of Veterans Affairs [VA], 2010). However, for some people, symptoms and cognitive deficits can persist for years (Ruff, 2005).

To understand the care received by nondeployed active-duty service members after an mTBI diagnosis, we analyzed individual-level health care utilization data. These administrative data detail when a service member visits a health care provider; characteristics of those visits, such as the location of care and the provider who treated the service member; the diagnoses and procedures that are recorded during those visits; and prescriptions filled by the service member. These data do not include clinical notes entered into the medical record by providers.

Military health care utilization data are managed and maintained by the Defense Health Agency, and the files used in our analysis were extracted from the MHS Data Repository. The repository contains records on all health care encounters paid for by the MHS; our analysis focused on health care use among nondeployed active-duty service members who received an mTBI diagnosis in calendar year 2012 and only health care received in garrison. We were not able to observe health care received in theater. The files were linked by scrambled Social Security numbers, so we were able to follow individual service members over time.

To augment the health care utilization data, we used individual-level data from the Defense Manpower Data Center (DMDC), which included the dates and locations of service members' deployments; service characteristics, such as rank and years of service; and dates of service, including separation date. These records were also linked by scrambled Social Security numbers, allowing us to match the identifiers in the Defense Health Agency data.

Drawing on these sources, we identified all active-component service members who had at least one health care encounter for an mTBI diagnosis in calendar year 2012. To do this, we first needed to select a case definition for mTBI. We conducted a search of the peer-reviewed and gray literature to identify existing case definitions for mTBI; compared the various existing definitions according to comprehensiveness, agreement, and other factors; and, in consultation with an expert advisory group, selected a working definition for the project. We also conducted analyses to determine the implications of selecting one definition over another.

The case definition for mTBI we selected is based on the ICD-9 and is used by the Armed Forces Health Surveillance Center. Using this definition, we examined the number of non-deployed active-duty service members who received treatment for an mTBI over five years (2008–2013), then compared our estimates to published DoD estimates of the number of service members with mTBI. We excluded National Guard and reserve service members from the analysis. It is likely that these service members have access to other health insurance, and we were not able to observe care that was not paid for by the MHS.

Figure S.1 shows the number of active-component service members who received treatment for an mTBI diagnosis between 2008 and 2013, according to our data. As shown in the figure, the number of service members who received treatment increased from 2008 to 2009 (from approximately 18,700 to nearly 22,000 cases), after which the number remained roughly steady through 2012.[1]

Characterizing Service Members Diagnosed with mTBI

We assessed the demographics, service history characteristics, and co-occurring conditions of the population of nondeployed active-duty service members who received treatment for a new mTBI in 2012, the most recent complete year of data at the time of this study. We defined a "new" mTBI as receipt of care associated with an mTBI diagnosis following a period of six months with no treatment for a TBI diagnosis.

We report sex, age, race/ethnicity, marital status, TRICARE region, branch of service, and rank, along with years of service and whether the service member had a history of deployments. We used DMDC data to determine whether a given service member had deployed since 2001;[2] those who had deployed since 2001 were characterized as having a "history of deployment." For characteristics that change over time (such as age), we report the value of the characteristic at the time of the first visit for the new mTBI.

---

[1]   TRICARE encounter data were extracted on or around October 24, 2013. Direct care data are considered complete within 90 days of an encounter; purchased care data are complete within 120 days. Therefore, we had access to complete direct and purchased care data through the end of June 2013. We extrapolated through the end of the calendar year to generate an estimate of 21,212 mTBI cases in 2013.

[2]   Our deployment data from DMDC's Contingency Tracking System included service members who were physically located in a designated combat zone or area of operation or who were specifically identified as directly supporting a deployment.

Figure S.1
Number of Nondeployed Active-Duty Service Members Who Received an mTBI Diagnosis, 2008–2013

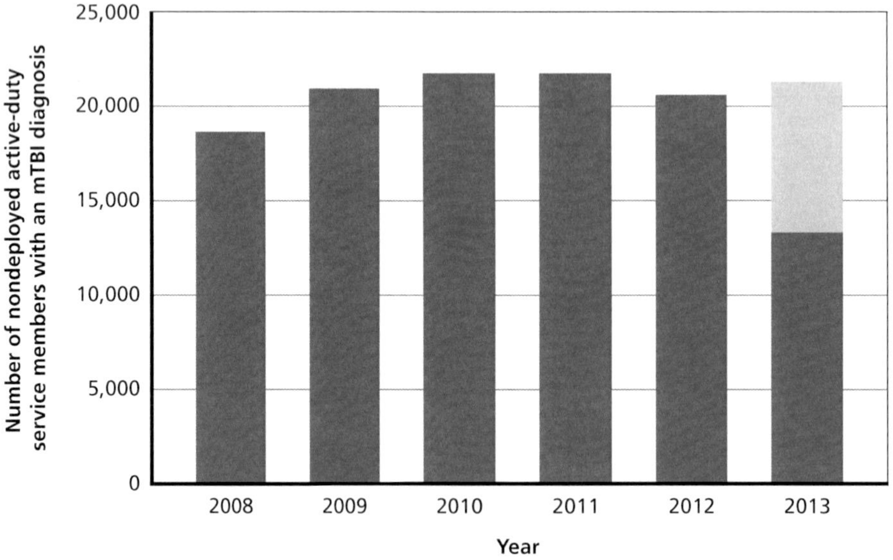

NOTE: Data through June 2013.
RAND RR844-S.1

Nondeployed Active-Duty Service Members with a New mTBI Tended to Be Young and Junior Enlisted

We found that nondeployed active-duty service members diagnosed with a new mTBI in 2012 tended to be relatively young and lower-ranked. Specifically, half of these service members were junior enlisted personnel at the time of diagnosis.[3] Service members with a new mTBI in 2012 had completed an average of six years of service, and two-thirds had a history of deployment. On average, those with a history of deployment had been deployed for 16 cumulative months prior to their 2012 mTBI diagnosis. These numbers varied by service, however, with Army personnel considerably more likely to have been deployed (79 percent), and for seven to nine months longer, than personnel from other service branches.

We also wanted to determine whether those service members with a new mTBI diagnosis in 2012 had previously received treatment for a TBI. Those who had received a TBI diagnosis of any severity in the years preceding the mTBI diagnosis in 2012 (i.e., between 2008 and 2011) were characterized as having a "history of TBI." We found that 10 percent of the 2012 mTBI cohort had received treatment for a previous TBI between 2008 and 2011.

Many Nondeployed Active-Duty Service Members with a New mTBI Received Treatment for Co-Occurring Behavioral Health Conditions, Pain, and Sleep Disorders

We used two methods to identify relevant co-occurring diagnoses in our study population. First, we reviewed the mTBI literature to develop a list of symptoms and conditions that occasionally or commonly occur as sequelae to mTBI (see, e.g., Borgaro et al., 2003; Lundin et al., 2006; Vaishnavi, Rao, and Fann, 2009).

---

[3]   See Cameron et al. (2012) for details on the link between junior rank and incidence of mTBI diagnosis.

Second, we examined the frequency of all ICD-9 codes associated with health care encounters in the six months following the first (diagnosis) visit for mTBI in our study population. Since service members may suffer other injuries as a consequence of the event that caused the mTBI, some of the symptoms and conditions we observed in the data may have been related to those injuries. We derived a subset of co-occurring conditions that were either commonly reported in the literature or frequently present in the mTBI cohort:

- *behavioral health conditions:* adjustment disorders, PTSD, other anxiety disorders (anxiety disorder not otherwise specified, panic disorder, generalized anxiety disorder), depression (major depressive disorder, dysthymia), acute stress disorders, bipolar disorder, delirium or dementia, attention deficit or attention deficit and hyperactivity disorder, alcohol abuse or dependence, and drug abuse or dependence
- *symptoms commonly or occasionally co-occurring with mTBI:* headache, other chronic pain, sleep disorders, irritability, memory loss, dizziness/vertigo, hearing problems, post-concussion syndrome, syncope and collapse, cognitive problems, skin sensation disturbances, alteration in mental status, gait and coordination problems, vision problems, communication disorders, and smell and taste disturbances.

We found that 11–16 percent of service members in the 2012 mTBI cohort received treatment for behavioral health conditions in the six months following their mTBI diagnosis, with adjustment disorders, anxiety disorders, depression, alcohol abuse/dependence, and PTSD the most common conditions for which service members received treatment. We observed that the mTBI diagnosis co-occurred with an increase in the proportion of service members who received treatment for behavioral health conditions; a smaller proportion (4–10 percent) received treatment for these conditions in the six months before mTBI diagnosis than in the six months after mTBI diagnosis.

In addition, in the six months following their mTBI diagnosis, many service members with a new mTBI received treatment for co-occurring headache (40 percent), back and neck pain (21 percent), and sleep disorders (25 percent). While some had received treatment for these conditions prior to the mTBI diagnosis (e.g., 12 percent had received treatment for back and neck pain in the six months before the mTBI diagnosis), for all conditions we examined, a higher proportion received treatment for these conditions after the mTBI diagnosis than before. We were also able to assess the clusters of diagnoses for these co-occurring conditions, finding that, for example, 68 percent of those who received treatment for headache also received treatment for a non-headache pain conditions and that 43 percent of those who received treatment for sleep disorders also received treatment for memory loss.

Analyzing Patterns of Care for Service Members Diagnosed with mTBI

Clinical research suggests that symptoms for most individuals with mTBI resolve within one month of the injury (Lundin et al., 2006; McCrea, Guskiewicz, et al., 2003). The symptoms and care of a small but not insignificant number of patients may persist to three months, and the symptoms of an even smaller group may persist for six months or longer. To ensure that we examined all potentially relevant care for every potential individual in our analysis, we selected an observation period of six months, though not all care observed during this time period was necessarily associated with the mTBI. We examined the clinical setting in which service members in the 2012 mTBI cohort received their mTBI diagnosis, the setting in which they had their next health care encounter, their patterns of health care use, and the types of assessments and treatments they received in the six months after the mTBI diagnosis.

Most Nondeployed Active-Duty Service Members with a New mTBI in 2012 Were Diagnosed in an Emergency Department and Had Their Next Health Care Visit in a Primary Care Setting

We characterized the treatment settings where service members in the mTBI cohort received care. We distinguished between *direct care*, which is care received at military treatment facilities (MTFs), and *purchased care*, which is care received in the community and paid for by TRICARE. We also identified whether the setting was a primary care clinic, emergency department, behavioral health specialty clinic, neurology clinic, inpatient facility, or other location.[4] In addition, we categorized the physical locations where service members in the mTBI cohort received care.

We found that 60 percent of the mTBI cohort was diagnosed in the direct care system; of these service members, 40 percent were diagnosed at a primary care clinic, and 35 percent received their diagnosis in an emergency department. Among the 40 percent who were diagnosed through the civilian purchased care network, the vast majority (80 percent) received their diagnosis in an emergency department. Thus, overall, half of all nondeployed active-duty service members with a new mTBI were diagnosed in an emergency department (see Figure S.2).

On average, service members in the 2012 mTBI cohort had their next health care encounter 17 days after the mTBI diagnosis, and these visits took place in the direct care system for 87 percent of the cohort. Nearly half of those visits took place in a primary care setting. Service

Figure S.2
Location of mTBI Diagnosis in the Direct and Purchased Care Systems

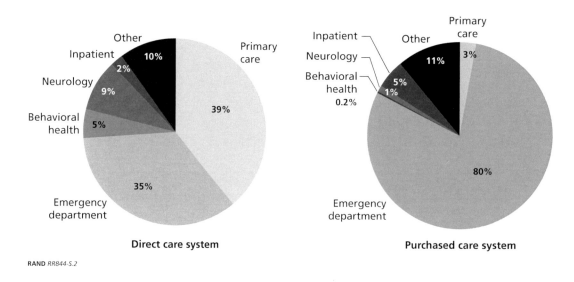

Direct care system

Purchased care system

---

[4] We were able to identify whether service members in the mTBI cohort received care from the Veterans Health Administration, but these cases accounted for fewer than 1 percent of the claims in our data.

members with a history of TBI or deployment were more likely to have their next health care encounter at a behavioral health clinic, compared with those without histories of deployment or TBI, who were more likely to be seen at a primary care clinic.

Most Nondeployed Active-Duty Service Members with mTBI Recovered Quickly

To identify patterns of care over the six-month time frame, we defined several time segments of treatment following the mTBI diagnosis, including treatment received within the first 24 hours and every week thereafter. We examined whether service members received any care (for any diagnosis or procedure), care potentially related to the mTBI (based on diagnosis codes for personal history of TBI), care for symptoms related to mTBI, and care for behavioral health diagnoses. Our findings agreed with the clinical research: The majority of service members in our cohort (80–90 percent) received care for three months or less following their initial mTBI diagnosis, with most (75–80 percent) receiving care for four weeks or less. However, a subset (10–20 percent) appeared to have persistent care needs—that is, they received ongoing mTBI-related care for longer than three months after the 2012 mTBI diagnosis.

Many Nondeployed Active-Duty Service Members with a New mTBI Received Diagnostic Assessments, Therapy, and Medications in the Six Months Following the mTBI Diagnosis, with Differences by TBI History

We identified diagnostic assessments, therapies, and medications potentially relevant to the treatment of common or occasional symptoms and conditions that can co-occur with mTBI using an approach similar to that described for comorbid diagnoses. First, we reviewed DoD/VA clinical practice guidelines (VA and DoD, 2009) for the treatment of mTBI and clinical guidance for the treatment of related symptoms (e.g., headache). We then developed a list of relevant assessments, therapies, and medications. We also reviewed the literature on the treatment of mTBI and consulted with an expert advisory group to identify additional relevant treatment. Finally, we examined the frequency of procedure codes (Current Procedural Terminology codes) associated with health care visits in the six months following the mTBI diagnostic visit, selecting those that were commonly received by the 202 mTBI cohort.

While we were not able to determine whether these were related to the mTBI or for another reason, the most common diagnostic assessments performed on nondeployed active-duty service members with a new mTBI were CT scans (33 percent), psychiatric diagnostic evaluations (28.7 percent), and physical therapy evaluations (24.8 percent). For almost every assessment or evaluation, service members with a history of TBI (any level of severity) were more likely than those without a history of TBI to receive these and other assessments and evaluations in the six months following their mTBI diagnosis.

The most frequently recommended initial treatment for mTBI is rest and patient education, activities that were not observable in our health care utilization data. However, many patients with mTBI receive care beyond the initial visit; as such, we report treatments received by the 2012 mTBI cohort in the six months following the mTBI diagnosis. We were not able to determine whether the care received was for the mTBI or for another condition, as current TBI coding guidance recommends that health care visits after the initial visit include symptom diagnostic codes rather than a TBI-related diagnostic code. As such, it is not possible to determine from these data whether physical therapy, for example, is related to the mTBI or a different condition.

Psychotherapy and physical therapy were the most common treatments received by the 2012 mTBI cohort in the six months following the mTBI diagnosis. As with diagnostic assessments, members of the cohort who experienced a prior TBI at the time of diagnosis were more likely to receive these treatments.

We also examined medication use, though, again, we were not able to attribute any filled prescriptions to the mTBI directly. We found that 60 percent of the cohort filled a prescription for analgesics in the six months following diagnosis, and half filled prescriptions for opioids; antidepressants were filled by one-quarter of the cohort. We observed that some had filled prescriptions for these medications prior to the mTBI diagnosis as well as after the diagnosis, indicating ongoing treatment for an unrelated condition (e.g., 15 percent filled a prescription for an opioid before and after the mTBI diagnosis), but the proportion who filled prescriptions for all medications we examined was higher after the mTBI diagnosis than before. Service members with a history of TBI at the time of their mTBI diagnosis were more likely to fill most types of prescriptions than were those without a history of TBI.

A Minority of Nondeployed Active-Duty Service Members with a New mTBI in 2012 Had Complex and Persistent Care Needs

We analyzed the characteristics and risk factors for those with persistent mTBI care needs. To identify potential risk factors among those needing persistent care, we calculated the adjusted relative risk for demographic characteristics and service history characteristics. Relative risk indicates the strength of the association between a characteristic and an outcome.

We identified 1,678 nondeployed active-duty service members with a new mTBI in 2012 who received mTBI-related treatment (indicated by a diagnosis of personal history of TBI) for longer than three months after the mTBI diagnosis ("persistent care"). We found that having a history of TBI was a significant risk factor for receiving persistent care following an mTBI diagnosis (see Table S.1). A service member was almost 50 percent more likely to receive persistent care if he or she had a previous TBI. We did not find a statistical relationship between sex and persistent care, contrary to findings from previous studies. We also found that those who had been deployed were two and a half times more likely to receive persistent care.

Strengths and Limitations of Our Approach

We used administrative health care utilization data for this analysis that captured medical care details for the population of nondeployed active-duty service members who received a new mTBI diagnosis in 2012. These data also included characteristics of the care they received following the mTBI diagnosis, including co-occurring diagnoses, procedures, medications, and the location and setting of care, as well as the demographic and service characteristics of individual patients. The data allowed us to describe health care utilization within a six-month period after an mTBI diagnosis and explore patterns of care that other data sources, such as surveys and reviews of medical records, would not allow.

Despite the comprehensiveness of these data, the analyses presented in this report have some limitations. First, we were not able to attribute care received after an mTBI diagnosis to the injury itself. This is because current coding guidance requires that the mTBI diagnostic code be recorded at the initial visit but not during subsequent visits. The coding guidance requires that providers record the diagnostic codes at subsequent visits for the chief complaint

Table S.1
Adjusted Relative Risk for Nondeployed Active-Duty Service Members Receiving Treatment 90 Days or More After mTBI Diagnosis, by Demographic Characteristics

Characteristic	2012 mTBI Cohort (n = 16,378)	Persistent Care (n = 1,678)		Adjusted Relative Risk
	Number	Number	%	
Sex				
Male	14,202	1,548	92.3	1.18
Female	2,176	130	7.7	0.85
Age at diagnosis				
18–34	14,018	1,352	80.6	0.75*
35 and older	2,360	326	19.4	1.33*
Race/ethnicity				
White, non-Hispanic	10,699	1,165	69.4	1.03
Black, non-Hispanic	2,319	190	11.3	0.79***
Hispanic	1,843	200	11.9	0.97
Other/unknown	1,517	123	7.3	1.14
Marital status				
Married	9,149	1,160	69.1	1.12
Never married	6,444	422	25.1	0.72***
Divorced/separated/widowed	778	96	5.7	1.24*
Region				
TRICARE North	4,421	431	25.8	1.14
TRICARE South	3,335	258	15.4	0.90
TRICARE West	6,930	821	49.1	1.26**
TRICARE Overseas	1,539	150	9.0	1.17
TBI history	1,611	294	17.5	1.48***
Service branch				
Army	8,791	1,306	77.8	3.75***
Navy	2,191	60	3.6	0.71
Air Force	2,686	46	2.7	0.41***
Marine Corps	2,248	261	15.6	3.74***
Other/unknown	462	5	0.3	0.25**
Deployment history	10,857	1,496	89.2	2.50***

NOTES: The relative risk is adjusted for gender, age, race, marital status, TRICARE region, TBI history, service branch, cumulative months of deployment, years of service, and deployment history. The analysis is based on health care encounters for personal history of TBI (ICD-9 code V15.52). Ninety days or more of treatment equates to persistent care. Numbers may not sum due to missing data.

*** Statistically significant difference at $p < 0.001$.
** Statistically significant difference at $p < 0.01$.
* Statistically significant difference at $p < 0.05$.

(e.g., headache), rather than the injury itself. This means that it was not possible to reliably determine whether subsequent assessments, treatments, or medications were part of mTBI treatment or unrelated to the mTBI.

Second, the data covered only care provided at MTFs and through the civilian purchased care network while service members were stationed in garrison. If a service member experienced an mTBI during a deployment, the data did not capture the initial diagnosis or any care received in theater. Relatedly, mTBI is often underdiagnosed (Powell et al., 2008); if service members received care for an mTBI but never received an mTBI diagnosis, that case would not be included in our data.

To identify diagnoses, we relied on ICD-9 diagnostic codes. In selecting and employing our ICD-9–based case definition of mTBI, we identified important issues related to the reliability and utility of this approach:

- *Prevalence estimates of mTBI are highly sensitive to case definitions.* Estimates of TBI are extremely sensitive to case definitions (AFHSC, 2009), and various definitions have been suggested for identifying TBI using ICD-9 diagnoses. This has resulted in a lack of easy comparability across research sources and settings.
- *Providers, within and across health care systems, are challenged by distinct and evolving coding guidance.* Patients move between military and civilian health care settings, where providers use unique coding rules for mTBI. Further, as understanding about mTBI has progressed since the start of the conflicts in Iraq and Afghanistan, guidance for mTBI coding has also evolved, resulting in multiple iterations of coding guidance within the past 15 years. For administrative codes to be applied consistently, there must be a shared understanding of how the codes are supposed to be applied. The rapid evolution of coding guidance and confusion among providers who work across health care systems are real challenges for the consistency of coding practices as it relates to mTBI.

Recommendations

1. Improve ICD-9 Coding Practices and Reconsider Current TBI Coding Guidance

Good administrative data should be considered integral to health care quality because these data help track the status of patients and the treatments and procedures they receive. DoD TBI coding guidance requires that providers record a TBI diagnosis only at the first visit, with subsequent visits coded with relevant symptom diagnostic codes rather than the TBI diagnostic code. As a result, it is not possible to use administrative data to observe treatment for mTBI over time. DoD should consider whether the advantages of the current TBI coding guidance outweigh the disadvantages for understanding the nature of care provided to service members with TBI.

2. Improve Data Quality to Increase Capacity for Research

The nature and purpose of administrative data pose real challenges for their use in research. Administrative data are collected for multiple purposes, including legal and financial reviews, that are largely unrelated to surveillance and research. This limits the data's utility for analysis. Improving connections between administrative claims and other clinical data (e.g., chart data, pharmacy data) is one way to enhance their value. The current lack of connectivity limits the use of the data for clinically relevant research. For example, it is often difficult to determine, using administrative data, whether referrals were followed up on or whether a prescription that was ordered was filled. Creating more interoperable data streams will facilitate a wide range of research.

3. Identify Opportunities to Coordinate Care

Our results demonstrate that nondeployed active-duty service members diagnosed with mTBI receive subsequent treatment in a variety of clinical settings. While not unique to mTBI, the specific challenges faced by these service members (and their providers) highlight the need for coordination of care and communication across providers, especially across direct- and purchased-care settings. It is important to understand current challenges and strategies for care coordination in this population and then identify best practices. Broader health system changes, such as the introduction of patient-centered care homes, may provide opportunities to coordinate care across provider types for service members with mTBI. Another approach could be to increase the role of the DVBIC Recovery Support Program or similar initiatives. The DVBIC recovery support specialists may be an effective means of enhancing coordination across providers, settings, and systems (Martin et al., 2013)

4. Assess Quality of Care for Service Members with mTBI

This report describes the types and patterns of care received by a cohort of service members with mTBI. However, our analyses were limited to variables available in an administrative data set, and we were unable to assess the quality of the care provided. Future efforts should extend our analysis to examine not only the type of care provided but also its quality. These studies will need to incorporate other data sources, as the administrative data do not include the details necessary to assess adherence to clinical practice guidelines. In addition, given the variability in symptom presentation and recovery, additional work is warranted to further develop standards of care for mTBI.

5. Extend These Results with Hypothesis-Driven, Multivariate Analyses

This study was designed to establish a foundation for hypothesis-directed clinical studies. To that end, we identified a number of areas that should be explored with further multivariate analyses to help the MHS confirm and interpret the relationships among patient, clinician, and setting factors in care patterns and outcomes for service members with mTBI. Multivariate regression can take multiple variables into account, helping to clarify when observed differences may be due to other factors. In particular, we recommend that future analyses focus on the following:

- *Examine co-occurring conditions and symptoms.* A number of co-occurring clinical conditions identified in our cohort should be considered for further examination. An extension of this research could involve factor analysis, cluster analysis, or other approaches that expand the scope from considering pairs of variables to considering multiple variables. If such clusters could be identified and account for a substantial portion of the variation in the original data, then these clusters might be useful for subsequent analyses, such as those regarding episodes of care. Such an endeavor would be complex, requiring substantial thought and care in conceptualizing these dependencies. It would likely require a novel conceptual model to rule out many contingencies and alternative explanations.

- *Explore predictors of care patterns.* Characterizing the course of care is a critical step in building statistical approaches to predicting it. The concept of a care episode, as used in this report, is one such approach, but specific inquiries could also examine particular aspects of the course of care. For example, does the course of care differ by diagnostic setting? Does the course of care differ for those who receive care from a TBI clinic? To what extent do variations in care patterns reflect differences in the initial severity of an mTBI?

- *Explore variation in care.* Our results offer some evidence of variation in care by service and history of TBI. Variation in care could reflect actual differences in the populations receiving treatment. MTFs and their providers could appropriately adjust their approach to diagnosis and treatment according to the unique needs of individual service members. Alternatively, variations in care could be associated with poorer quality of care. Understanding the reasons for observed differences can inform quality improvement initiatives and reduce inappropriate variations in care.

- *Examine a clinical cohort with persistent mTBI-related problems.* Some service members have persistent mTBI care needs. To address these needs, improved understanding of this group is required. As a first step, it will be important to accurately identify service members who have ongoing care needs and to further understand the risk factors associated with persistent care. While administrative data allowed us to examine persistent care among the population of service members with mTBI, there are the limitations to this approach, most notably issues associated with proper diagnostic coding. Other data sources, such as clinical data or medical record data, would help in better identifying service members with long-term needs.

Concluding Thoughts

As a signature injury of modern warfare, TBI affects more service members than ever before. Mild TBI, the most common TBI severity, can be challenging to identify and treat due to variations in symptom presentation and other factors. This report presents information to answer questions about how many and which service members receive an mTBI diagnosis, where they receive care, the types of treatment they receive, and for how long they receive care. The important baseline information presented here is a key step toward the ultimate goal of providing high-quality care for service members receiving treatment for mTBI in the MHS.

Acknowledgments

We gratefully acknowledge the support of our current and previous project sponsors, Elisabeth Moy Martin and CDR Kathleen Grudzien, as well as the staff at the Defense and Veterans Brain Injury Center, particularly Dorothy Kaplan.

We also thank the members of our expert advisory group: Carolyn Caldwell, U.S. Army, Northern Region Medical Command; Timothy Camasta, Warrior Recovery Center, Fort Carson, Colorado; CDR Vincent DeCicco, Health Services, Headquarters, U.S. Marine Corps; Daniel Evatt, Defense Health Clinical Center, Defense Centers of Excellence for Psychological Health and Traumatic Brain Injury; Brian Ivins, Defense and Veterans Brain Injury Center; CAPT Thomas Johnson, Intrepid Spirit Concussion Recovery Center, Camp Lejeune, North Carolina; James Kelly, National Intrepid Center of Excellence; Lt Col Jeffrey Lewis, U.S. Air Force; Donald W. Marion, Defense and Veterans Brain Injury Center; CDR Renee Pazdan, Warrior Recovery Center, Fort Carson, Colorado; Lemma E. Regasa, Defense and Veterans Brain Injury Center; Leigh Selby, U.S. Army Europe Regional Medical Command; Gary Southwell, U.S. Army Western Regional Medical Command; and CAPT Jack Tsao, U.S. Navy Bureau of Medicine and Surgery. The input provided by this group was invaluable and informed the analyses, interpretations, and recommendations described in this report. Members of this group are not responsible for the contents of this report or the recommendations contained herein.

We appreciate the valuable insights we received from Lisa Brenner and Susan Straus. We addressed their constructive critiques as part of RAND's rigorous quality assurance process to improve the quality of this report. We thank Lauren Skrabala for her writing and editing support and Tiffany Hruby, Cate Yoon, and Diane Egelhoff for their assistance in preparing this report.

Abbreviations

ADD	attention deficit disorder
ADHD	attention deficit hyperactivity disorder
AFHSC	Armed Forces Health Surveillance Center
BiPAP	bilevel positive airway pressure
CAM	complementary and alternative medicine
CDC	Centers for Disease Control and Prevention
CPAP	continuous positive airway pressure
CPT	Current Procedural Terminology
CT	computed tomography
DCoE	Defense Centers of Excellence for Psychological Health and Traumatic Brain Injury
DHA	Defense Health Agency
DMDC	Defense Manpower Data Center
DoD	U.S. Department of Defense
DVBIC	Defense and Veterans Brain Injury Center
ICD	International Classification of Diseases
IED	improvised explosive device
MHS	Military Health System
MRI	magnetic resonance imaging
mTBI	mild traumatic brain injury
MTF	military treatment facility
NSAID	nonsteroidal anti-inflammatory drug
OCD	obsessive-compulsive disorder

OEF   Operation Enduring Freedom

OIF   Operation Iraqi Freedom

PCS   post-concussion syndrome

PTSD   post-traumatic stress disorder

TBI   traumatic brain injury

VA   U.S. Department of Veterans Affairs

VHA   Veterans Health Administration

CHAPTER ONE

Introduction

The number of service members diagnosed with a traumatic brain injury (TBI) has increased in recent years (Defense and Veterans Brain Injury Center [DVBIC], 2014a). This is due in part to the large number of service members (approximately 2.5 million) who deployed to Iraq and Afghanistan between 2001 and 2013. A survey published in 2008 found that nearly 20 percent of service members who had deployed to those conflict zones reported an injury during their most recent deployment that resulted in a loss of consciousness (Schell and Marshall, 2008). The costs associated with these injuries can be substantial. One estimate, based on a microsimulation model, suggested that the total cost of deployment-related TBIs was between $591 million and $910 million (in 2007 dollars; Eibner et al., 2008).

Deployment-related injuries are not the only driver of TBIs, however. Outside of deployment injuries, service members are at higher risk of TBIs than civilian populations (Warden, 2006). These injuries may result from a range of activities, including training accidents, accidental falls, sports-related concussions, and motor vehicle accidents (Logan et al., 2013). Non–deployment-related TBIs accounted for 84 percent of all TBIs reported to the U.S. Department of Defense (DoD) between 2001 and 2011 (Office of the Surgeon General, 2013).

While the number of TBIs has been growing among military service personnel, the number identified and diagnosed with TBI in the Military Health System (MHS) has also increased. The annual number of active-duty service members diagnosed with TBI by a medical professional grew from 12,470 in 2002 to a peak of 32,668 in 2011 (DVBIC, 2014a). The reasons for the increase in TBI diagnoses could be attributable to a variety of factors including those that are deployment-related, such as an increase in improvised explosive device (IED) attacks, combat approach (e.g., the 2007 troop "surge" in Iraq), or factors unrelated to deployment, such as an increase in population-based screening and increased provider recognition of TBI (Logan et al., 2013).

Diagnostic Criteria for Mild Traumatic Brain Injury

TBI is defined as "a blow or jolt to the head or a penetrating head injury that disrupts the function of the brain" (DVBIC, 2014b). Injuries can be penetrating or non-penetrating, with non-penetrating injuries involving a force, fall, or blow that causes the brain to be compressed against the walls of the skull or experience other mechanical forces causing injury. Damage can result from blood vessel hemorrhages, neuronal death, shearing of axonal fibers, a secondary inflammatory cascades and other factors. TBI varies in severity, and is characterized as mild, moderate, and severe *at the time of the injury*. Table 1.1 highlights the differences between

Table 1.1
DoD/VA Common Classifications of TBI Severity

Mild TBI	Moderate TBI	Severe TBI
Normal structural imaging, CT scan	Normal or abnormal structural imaging, CT scan	Normal or abnormal structural imaging, CT scan
Loss of consciousness for less than 30 minutes	Loss of consciousness for more than 30 minutes and less than 24 hours	Loss of consciousness more than 24 hours
Alteration of consciousness for one moment up to 24 hours	Alteration of consciousness for more than 24 hours	Alteration of consciousness for more than 24 hours
Post-traumatic amnesia for 1 day or less	Post-traumatic amnesia for more than 1 and less than 7 days	Post-traumatic amnesia for more than 7 days
Glasgow Coma Scale = 13–15	Glasgow Coma Scale = 9–12	Glasgow Coma Scale = 3–8

SOURCE: Defense Centers of Excellence for Psychological Health and Traumatic Brain Injury (DCoE) and DVBIC, 2010.

NOTES: The Glasgow Coma Scale is a clinical method used to rate a patient's level of consciousness on a combination of three tests: eye response, verbal response, and motor response. A combined score of 3 represents a severe brain injury and 15 represents a very mild injury or full consciousness.

severity levels of TBI, using criteria established by DoD and the U.S. Department of Veterans Affairs (VA).

Mild TBI (mTBI), also known as concussion, is typically invisible to current clinical MRI or CT technology, whereas individuals with moderate and severe TBI tend to have abnormal MRI or CT scans (Hoge, Goldberg, and Castro, 2009). Other indicators of mTBI following a trauma include little to no loss of consciousness (less than 30 minutes), an altered mental state lasting less than 24 hours, and amnesia lasting less than 24 hours. In contrast, moderate and severe TBI can be marked by a loss of consciousness lasting longer than 30 minutes, an altered mental state lasting longer than 24 hours, amnesia that persists for days (moderate) or weeks (severe), and impaired motor, verbal, and eye-opening responses.

Typical symptoms of moderate and severe TBI are quite observable and include persistent headache, vomiting or nausea, convulsions or seizures, coma or vegetative state, dilation of one or both pupils, dysfunctional speech, weakness or numbness in the extremities, loss of coordination, and increased confusion, restlessness, or agitation (National Institue of Neurological Disorders and Stroke, 2014). In contrast, common symptoms of mTBI, which include headache, confusion, irritability, aggression, and memory and concentration difficulties, are often associated with other conditions or dismissed as transitory, making identification and appropriate diagnosis challenging (VA, 2010; DVBIC Working Group on Acute Management of Mild Traumatic Brain Injury in Military Operational Settings, 2006; McCrea, Iverson, et al., 2009). Particularly in military populations, mTBI has often been confounded with other trauma-related disorders, such as post-traumatic stress disorder (PTSD; Bryant, 2010), as both conditions are associated with experiencing a traumatic event. As expected, evidence suggests that veterans who have experienced injuries that could be classified as TBIs may be more likely to report PTSD symptoms when compared with veterans who have not experienced an injury event or TBI symptoms (Hoge, Goldberg, and Castro, 2009).

While the severity of the TBI at the time of the acute injury has some prognostic value, the course of symptom improvement following injury can vary widely (VA, 2010). For patients with a moderate or severe TBI, long-term outcomes can vary from full recovery to complete dependence on care providers. Measurable deficits in cognitive and physical functioning may still exist a year after the injury (Andelic et al., 2010; Novack et al., 2000). In contrast, symptoms associated with mTBI tend to resolve quickly for the majority of patients. Existing studies suggest that the majority of symptoms tend to resolve within the first month after an mTBI incident (Lundin et al., 2006; McCrea, Guskiewicz, et al., 2003), with cognitive symptoms largely resolving after three months. However, some people experience symptoms and cognitive deficits that continue for years (Ruff, 2005).

Why Focus on Mild TBI Among Service Members?

DVBIC asked RAND to assess care provided to service members with an mTBI diagnosis. Although patients with mTBI have experienced a less severe injury event, they remain a large, high-priority population. According to DVBIC annual reporting, mTBIs represent 84 percent of all TBIs among service members, while more severe TBIs (including moderate, severe, and penetrating) account for around 8 percent (DVBIC, 2014a).[1] These data suggest that many more service members will be affected by mTBI than by moderate or severe TBI. Further, appropriate identification and diagnosis of mTBI may be more challenging due to the limited validity of diagnostic tools for mTBI (e.g., CT scans and cognitive testing) (Borg et al., 2004) and symptoms that overlap with those of other conditions (e.g., PTSD, depression; Borg et al., 2004; Hoge, McGurk, et al., 2008). In addition, patients with mTBI may have varying courses of treatment, depending on the severity of subsequent symptoms and their resolution (DVBIC, 2014c; DCoE and DVBIC, 2010). The health care costs associated with mTBI have not been studied in the military, but a civilian study found that costs for non–mental health care among people with mTBI were 75 percent higher than in a matched sample without TBI, and the difference grew to almost double if a person with an mTBI had a comorbid psychiatric disorder (Rockhill et al., 2012).

This is the first comprehensive analysis of the care delivered by the MHS to nondeployed active-duty service members who have experienced an mTBI. The findings capture the characteristics of all nondeployed active-duty service members who received an mTBI diagnosis through the MHS in 2012, their symptoms and co-occurring conditions, and the location, type, and duration of care they received.

Understanding the Care Provided by the Military Health System for mTBI

There are several unanswered questions about the characteristics of service members who receive treatment for mTBI through the MHS, the types of they care receive, and course of their care. Challenges in accurately diagnosing an mTBI make it difficult to consistently identify patients who receive care for the condition and to characterize the usual care for these patients (Helmick et al., 2012; Hoge, McGurk, et al., 2008). Further, there has been little research on the course of symptoms and treatment pathways for mTBI. This has led researchers to call for a better understanding of the natural history of the condition, including patterns of care received (Laborde, 2000; Manley and Maas, 2013). Identifying patterns of care could

[1]   The remaining 9 percent of TBIs are "not classifiable."

inform improved approaches to prevention, methods to minimize the negative impact on both the service member and the force, strategies for improving recovery, and the development of standards of care.

The purpose of this report is to describe the characteristics of the population of nondeployed active-duty service members who were diagnosed with mTBI through the MHS and to describe the care they received following diagnosis using health care utilization data. The goal of our analysis was to fill some of the gaps in understanding regarding the usual care for this condition and to lay the groundwork for future research to assess and improve the quality of care.

Figure 1.1 shows the three overarching analytic goals addressed in this report. First, we evaluated multiple methods of identifying service members with mTBI using diagnostic codes. Appropriate identification and diagnosis of mTBI is challenging, but clinicians also vary in their approach to diagnostic coding for TBI. Second, we compiled and reviewed data on the population characteristics of those who were diagnosed with mTBI, along with the types of care received, the settings in which care was provided, and the types of providers who delivered the care. Finally, we explored patterns of care among those diagnosed with mTBI. We determined the duration of care and identified patterns of utilization. In addition, we reviewed data on service members who received "persistent care," defined as care received beyond three months after the injury.

To understand the care received by service members diagnosed with mTBI, we analyzed individual-level health care utilization data. These administrative data detail when a service member visited a health care provider; characteristics of those visits, such as the location of care and the provider who treated the service member; the diagnoses and procedures recorded during those visits; and prescriptions filled by the service member. While these data can include postdeployment care for mTBI, they do not capture diagnoses and health care delivered in theater. As such, our analyses focus on nondeployed service members who received care through the MHS.

Strengths and Limitations of Using Administrative Data to Describe Care Following an mTBI Diagnosis

The administrative data used for our analyses included data on every visit for every service member at military treatment facilities (MTFs) and in the civilian sector, paid for by

Figure 1.1
Overview of Approach to Describing Care Following mTBI Diagnosis

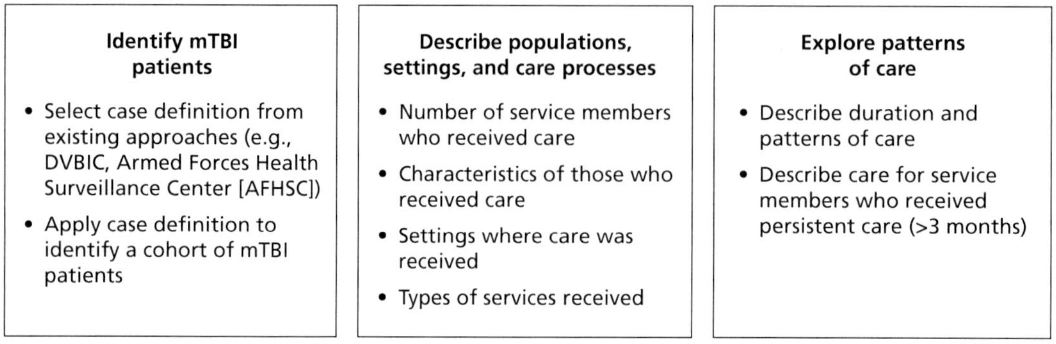

Identify mTBI patients	Describe populations, settings, and care processes	Explore patterns of care
• Select case definition from existing approaches (e.g., DVBIC, Armed Forces Health Surveillance Center [AFHSC]) • Apply case definition to identify a cohort of mTBI patients	• Number of service members who received care • Characteristics of those who received care • Settings where care was received • Types of services received	• Describe duration and patterns of care • Describe care for service members who received persistent care (>3 months)

TRICARE, the health insurance provider for active-duty service members. No other data source (e.g., medical records, patient surveys, provider surveys) allows for such a comprehensive examination of *all care provided by the MHS*. Alternative data sources must rely on selecting and inferring from a sample. The analyses of administrative data presented in this report characterize many aspects of care and highlight where other data sources and approaches could be useful in subsequent work to more fully identify ways to improve care for mTBI. While the limitations described here suggest the need for some caution when interpreting the results, there are limitations associated with alternative data sources as well.

First, identifying patients with mTBI can be challenging, regardless of data source. As noted earlier, there is significant variation among clinicians in their approaches to identifying and diagnosing mTBI. When describing care using administrative data, we were able to observe care only for patients who had been diagnosed with mTBI. This condition is often underdiagnosed (Powell et al., 2008); if service members received care for an mTBI, yet never received an mTBI diagnosis, we could not observe that care.

Relatedly, clinicians vary in their use of diagnosis codes for mTBI. In this report, we focus primarily on nondeployed active-duty service members with new diagnoses of mTBI. Coding guidance suggests that the diagnostic code for a new TBI in the International Classification of Diseases, Ninth Revision (ICD-9), Clinical Modification, should be used only at the first detection of the condition (TRICARE, undated; DoD, 2010). Yet, patients may be seen in multiple settings and may have several visits in which different clinicians use this "first" diagnosis. Alternatively, clinicians may either miss the opportunity to the use the "first" diagnosis or repeat it several times. In conducting this study, we assumed that patients' mTBI diagnoses and related administrative codes are accurate. Appendix A offers an in-depth discussion of the challenges in identifying mTBI through administrative data and how those challenges applied to this study.

Describing mTBI-related care is also challenging. Coding guidelines suggest the use of V-codes, or history of injury codes (e.g., V15.52, history of TBI; DoD, 2010), to link care that is associated with an mTBI diagnosis to subsequent visits. In practice, these codes may be used inconsistently. For example, the V-code may not be attached to the primary diagnosis visit, or it may be absent from any mTBI-related visit. In addition, some care provided to patients with mTBI, such as sleep hygiene, is not recorded in administrative data because there is not an associated procedure code for this type of service. Interventions that are only documented by the provider in the clinical note in the medical record are not captured. Thus, findings from the administrative data are limited in their ability to directly inform clinical practice guidelines. Follow-up work that examines clinical notes in the medical record could more directly inform practice guidelines, along with additional efficacy trials to identify evidence-based interventions.

Finally, characterizing duration and patterns of care related to an mTBI diagnosis can also be challenging. Symptoms associated with mTBI resolve quickly for most patients but may linger for some time for others. Routine outcome monitoring of symptoms is uncommon in the administrative data, so tracking the clinical course and response to treatment for a particular patient is usually not possible. Therefore, we were limited to selecting a time window (e.g., six months after initial injury) and characterizing the receipt and patterns of care over that period.

Despite these limitations, this is likely the most comprehensive assessment of care provided to service members with mTBI ever conducted. The findings presented in this report fill some of the gaps in understanding regarding usual care for this condition and lay the groundwork for future research to assess and improve the quality of that care.

Organization of This Report

The remainder of this report describes our methodological approach and the results of our analyses and concludes with recommendations. Chapter Two provides a description of our approach to selecting a case definition of mTBI, along with an overview of our analyses. Chapter Three describes the number of service members who received care for mTBI. Subsequently, in Chapter Four, we describe the characteristics of these service members, including demographic and military service characteristics and their co-occurring conditions and associated symptoms. Chapter Five examines where service members receive care, both for their initial mTBI diagnosis and for follow-up care. Chapter Six profiles mTBI episodes of care, including the duration of treatment for mTBI and patterns of care for those with a new mTBI. In Chapter Seven, we describe diagnostic evaluations and assessments and various treatments provided, including therapies and medications. Finally, in Chapter Eight, we describe care for service members who received treatment for mTBI symptoms three months or more after their injury. We conclude with a summary of our findings and recommendations in Chapter Nine.

Five appendixes provide additional detail on the use of diagnostic (ICD-9) codes to identify mTBI cases (Appendix A), a comparison of our selected case definition of mTBI with other published definitions (Appendix B), and considerations to account for in shifting from ICD-9 to ICD-10 codes (Appendix C). Appendix D offers additional methodological detail on how variables were defined, and Appendix E presents additional analyses to support our findings regarding treatment and location of treatment by service, deployment history, TBI history, and history of treatment for co-occurring conditions.

CHAPTER TWO

Methods

In this chapter, we first provide an overview of our methodology. Then, we describe the data sources and our approach to identifying a cohort of service members with a new diagnosis of mTBI. We define the variables that we used to describe the characteristics of these service members and the care they received. We conclude with a discussion of our approach to defining and characterizing episodes of care.

Overview

As described in Chapter One, the goal of this study was to describe the characteristics of the population of nondeployed active-duty service members who received treatment for an mTBI through the MHS, along with the location and types of care they received. We consulted with an expert advisory group made up of TBI experts and researchers who provided feedback and guidance on our analyses.

There were three phases to our analysis (see Table 2.1). First, we needed to select a case definition for mTBI that could be applied to health care utilization data. We conducted a search of the peer-reviewed and gray literature to identify existing case definitions for mTBI; compared the various existing definitions according to comprehensiveness, agreement, and other factors; and, in consultation with the expert advisory group, selected a working definition for the project. We also conducted analyses to determine the implications of selecting one definition over another.

Second, we developed an approach to defining an episode of care for common or occasional symptoms and conditions that can co-occur with mTBI, beginning with identifying a new mTBI case and determining the appropriate duration of follow-up care after the initial visit. As we describe later, using administrative data to characterize mTBI care is not straightforward, so we developed an approach based on the nature and timing of care relative to the mTBI diagnosis for common and occasional symptoms and conditions that can co-occur with an mTBI. We also examined patterns of care to determine the length of a typical episode. Finally, we identified the subpopulation with persistent care needs and assessed the risk factors for needing such care.

Table 2.1
Analysis Steps

Phase and Step	Description
Develop a Case Definition for mTBI	
1	Identify alternative case definitions for mTBI
2	Develop coding strategy for each alternative
3	Choose one of the alternative definitions
Assess Patterns of Care	
4	Identify types of care that are potentially attributable to common or occasional symptoms and conditions that can co-occur with mTBI
5	Identify a length of time over which potentially attributable care will be provided
6	Examine patterns of care
Describe Persistent Care for Common or Occasional Symptoms and Conditions That Can Co-Occur with mTBI	
7	Identify alternative definitions for persistent care
8	Develop coding strategy for each alternative
9	Choose alternative definitions for persistent care
10	Examine persistent care after mTBI diagnosis

Expert Advisory Group

To inform our analyses, we convened a group of 14 experts in the treatment of mTBI in the context of the MHS. This expert advisory group included representatives from across DoD. The study team met with the group three times by teleconference and web meeting over the course of this study. During these meetings, we presented our proposed approaches to developing the mTBI case definition and analyzing episodes of care, and we presented our preliminary findings. We solicited and incorporated the group members' feedback on the mTBI case definition and the presentation of results. We note that while the expert advisory group informed this project, the members were not asked to approve the final report and, hence, are not responsible for this report or its contents.

Data Sources

To characterize the treatment of mTBI, we used individual-level health care utilization data. These data detail when a service member visits a health care provider; characteristics of those visits, such as the location of care and the provider who treated the service member; the diagnoses and procedures recorded during those visits; and prescriptions filled by the service member. The data do not include clinical notes entered into the medical record by providers.

Military health care utilization data are managed and maintained by the Defense Health Agency (DHA), and the specific files used in this analysis were extracted from the MHS Data Repository. The data contain records on all health care encounters paid for by the MHS, and our extract covered health care use from fiscal year 2008 through June 2013. All files in the repository were linked to individuals by scrambled Social Security numbers, so we were able to follow individual service members over time.

The DHA data captured health care utilization in two related systems of care: direct and purchased care. Care that is delivered in MTFs is called *direct care*, and although TRICARE does not pay directly for care that is provided by MTFs, information about health care visits is recorded as if these were claims paid by an insurance provider. If an MTF is unable to provide the care a service member needs due to capacity or capability constraints, the service member will be referred to a civilian provider in the TRICARE network. Care that is delivered in this way is called *purchased care*. The DHA data that we used in this analysis included any patient encounter with a network civilian provider for which the MHS was a payer.[1] In addition to inpatient and outpatient encounters on the direct and purchased care networks, the data contained information about medications filled by the patient.

To augment the DHA health care utilization data, we used data from the Defense Manpower Data Center (DMDC), which included the dates and locations of service members' deployments; service characteristics, such as rank and years of service; and dates of service, including separation date, when formerly active-component service members become ineligible for TRICARE-covered health care. These were also individual-level data, with scrambled Social Security numbers matching the identifiers in the DHA data.

Population

We identified all nondeployed active-duty service members who received treatment for a new mTBI in calendar year 2012. We defined mTBI using ICD-9 codes, as described in the next section. We excluded service members who were in the National Guard or reserve because these service members may have access to VA and other health insurance, and we would not have been able to observe the care that they received that was not paid for by the MHS.

Selecting a Case Definition for mTBI

Health care utilization data include variables that describe the diagnoses recorded during a health care encounter and the treatment that was delivered. Diagnoses are recorded according to the International Classification of Diseases (ICD). During the period of our analysis, the ninth revision, clinical modification, was in use (National Center for Health Statistics, 2013).[2] To identify which service members received treatment for mTBI, we first needed to use ICD-9 codes to define a "case" of TBI and, specifically, mild TBI.

---

[1] If the service member had other insurance, such as through a spouse's employer, and the MHS did not pay for the health care encounter, we were not able to determine the care that was delivered.

[2] While some health care systems and providers are transitioning (or have transitioned) to the ICD-10, TRICARE follows the official guidelines put forward by the U.S. Department of Health and Human Services. The department issued a final rule to transition to the ICD-10 on October 1, 2015, well after these analyses were conducted. However, Appendix C notes how the definitions used in our analyses compare with possible ICD-10 definitions (U.S. Department of Health and Human Services, 2014).

Our first step was to conduct a broad-based literature review, informally weighting studies according to four primary criteria:

1. The study's definition had be administrative-data based.
2. The case definitions were widely used.
3. The case definitions focused on the military population.
4. The case definitions focused on mTBI, though we considered general TBI case definitions as well.

Second, we selected a number of definitions from the literature, plus one narrow definition focusing only on concussion.[3] We then compared the included ICD-9 codes across several code categories. From this comparison exercise (Appendix B), we created three proposed case definitions for mTBI, which varied the population captured by the definition, as well as the literature reflected (i.e., military- or civilian-oriented).

Next, we presented the three proposed case definitions to our expert advisory group. The group provided feedback that helped us tailor an approach centering on the DoD definition of mTBI, the case definition in use by the DVBIC and AFHSC and shown in Table 2.2 (AFHSC, 2012). The primary reasons for the definition's selection were (1) its applicability to the military population, (2) its consistency with current military coding practice toward cap-

Table 2.2
DVBIC/AFHSC Case Definition for mTBI

ICD Code Group	Description
850	Concussion (850.0, 850.11, 850.5, 850.9)
800.0	Closed fracture of vault of skull (800.00, 800.01, 800.02, 800.06, 800.09)
800.5	Open fracture of vault of skull (800.50, 800.51, 800.52)
801.0	Closed fracture of base of skull (801.00, 801.01, 801.02, 801.06, 801.09)
801.5	Open fracture of base of skull (801.50, 801.51, 801.52)
803.0	Other closed skull fracture (803.00, 803.01, 803.02, 803.06, 803.09)
803.5	Other open skull fracture (803.50, 803.51, 803.52)
804.0	Closed fractures involving skull or face with other bones (804.00, 804.01, 804.02, 804.06, 804.09)
804.5	Open fractures involving skull or face with other bones (804.50, 804.51, 804.52)
950 and 959	Other head injury (959.01)
310	Postconcussion syndrome (310.2)
V15.52	Personal history of TBI (current standard; 2010–the time of this research)*

NOTE: More detailed codes are presented in Appendix A.

* This code reflects current DoD coding guidance, updated in 2010. Prior to this time, other codes were used to capture TBI history. However, these codes were less targeted, and, while coding practice may vary, we made the decision to use the more specific code.

[3] See National Center for Injury Prevention and Control, 2003; Faul et al., 2010; "Incident Diagnoses of Common Symptoms," 2013; Coronado et al., 2011; AFHSC, 2012; Wojcik et al., 2010; Bazarian et al., 2006; and MacGregor et al., 2010.

turing a broader population, and (3) its widespread use in the gray and academic literature, for ease of comparisons. This case definition has been used by DVBIC and AFHSC for surveillance purposes and was established in 2008 by an expert working group using an AFHSC-developed process for case definition. The definition is updated periodically; we used the most current version at the time of our research, which had most recently been revised in 2010 (AFHSC, 2013).

We were also aware from the literature (AFHSC, 2009) and feedback from our expert advisory group that the project results could be highly sensitive to the case definition. In Appendix B, we make comparisons between the DVBIC/AFHSC case definition used in this report and other major definitions and discuss how definition variations could affect the study's results.

To assess the robustness of the case definition we selected, we examined the number of nondeployed active-duty service members who received treatment for an mTBI between 2008 and 2013 and compared our estimates to published DoD estimates of the number of service members with mTBI.[4]

Identifying Service Members with a New mTBI

Our analysis of mTBI treatment focused on calendar year 2012, the most recent for which we had a complete year of data. We examined care for all nondeployed active-duty service members who were diagnosed with an mTBI in 2012, though we note that these service members may have sustained and been diagnosed with a previous mTBI prior to that period.

DoD ICD-9 coding guidance stipulates that diagnostic codes for TBI should be recorded during the initial health care encounter for the injury but not during subsequent visits. Subsequent visits should instead include ICD-9 diagnostic codes for the chief complaint (e.g., headache, sleep problems), along with a secondary diagnostic code to indicate a personal history of TBI (V15.52; TRICARE, undated; DoD, 2010).

In following this guidance, most of the ICD-9 codes included in the DVBIC/AFHSC case definition for mTBI can be used to identify a new mTBI. There are two exceptions, however: The DVBIC/AFHSC case definition includes personal history of TBI (V15.52) and post-concussion syndrome (PCS, 310.2), both of which are diagnostic codes used to indicate treatment for a previous TBI, not a new injury. PCS, by definition, is not typically diagnosed until three or more months after an injury.[5] Therefore, we excluded these codes when identifying a new mTBI.

It is likely that there is variation in the extent to which providers across the MHS adhere to the DoD ICD-9 coding guidance (Lloyd and Rissing, 1985). For example, many providers may record the mTBI diagnostic code during subsequent visits rather than only during the initial visit; this is common coding practice for most other diagnoses (TRICARE, undated). To better ensure that we were capturing new mTBI diagnoses only and not treatment for a previous mTBI, we restricted our analyses to cases in which service members did not have any

---

[4] Treatment for mTBI is based on ICD-9 identification of mTBI, assuming that the diagnosis and coding accurately portray the service member's condition. Further discussion of the limitations of administrative data can be found in Appendix A.

[5] Personal history of TBI and PCS are included in the DVBIV/AFHSC case definition for surveillance purposes, as it is possible that there was no prior documentation of the injury for the patient (i.e., the coding for personal history of injury or PCS may be recorded as the first instance of a TBI-related visit).

health care encounters coded with a TBI diagnosis of any severity in the previous six months (a "clean period"), followed by a health care encounter with an mTBI diagnostic code (the "diagnosis visit"), as shown in Figure 2.1. We then analyzed the care that was received in the six months following the initial mTBI diagnosis.

We further restricted our analyses to only those service members who were eligible for TRICARE benefits for the 12 months of our analysis period (i.e., the six-month clean period and six-month observation period). Because we focused on active-duty service members, we assumed that they were eligible for care through the MHS as long as they were serving in that capacity. Therefore, we used the date of separation from the military to define their eligibility and included in our analysis only those service members who did not separate within six months of their mTBI diagnosis.

Using these criteria, we identified 16,378 service members who received treatment for a new mTBI in calendar year 2012 (hereafter, the 2012 mTBI cohort).

Analyses

Descriptive Analyses

The primary purpose of our analysis was to describe the landscape of care for nondeployed active-duty service members who received treatment for a new mTBI in 2012. We identified the number and characteristics of the population of service members who received treatment following a new mTBI diagnosis in 2012, as well as the locations and treatment settings where they received their diagnosis and had their first-follow up visit. We also reviewed the types of assessments and treatments that were received by this population, for whatever cause, in the six months following their mTBI diagnosis.

In Chapters Three through Eight, we present results for the entire mTBI cohort and analyze differences according to the presence or absence of a history of TBI (i.e., whether a service member in the 2012 mTBI cohort received treatment for another TBI of any severity in the three years prior to 2012). Based on prior research, we expected that service members with a history of TBI would be more likely to have co-occurring health problems (e.g., Schatz et al., 2011; Spira et al., 2014; Stein and McAllister, 2009) and to receive a wide range of medical, behavioral health, rehabilitation, and specialty care (Lew, Otis, et al., 2009; Lew, Pogoda, et al., 2011; Taylor et al., 2012). We present differences by service branch and deployment history in Appendix E. We used administrative data to determine whether the service member had been deployed since 2001 and prior to a diagnosis of mTBI. Deployments in this setting are defined as a service member being physically located in a designated combat zone or area of

Figure 2.1
Analysis of Care for a New mTBI

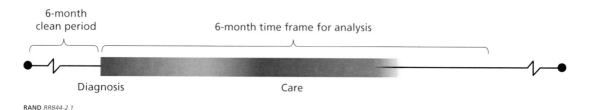

operations or when a member has specifically been identified by his or her service as directly supporting deployments to Iraq or Afghanistan. For each of these comparisons, we conducted t-tests (differences by TBI history and deployment history) or chi-square tests (differences by service) and indicate which differences are statistically significant (p < 0.05). Throughout, the reader should keep in mind that some results on these statistical tests will be significant simply by chance.

Patterns of Care

Clinical research suggests that symptoms for most patients resolve within one month of the mTBI-linked injury (Lundin et al., 2006; McCrea, Guskiewicz, et al., 2003). However, it is not possible using an administrative data set to identify in advance patients for whom a one-month resolution can be expected. The symptoms and care of a small but not insignificant number of patients may persist for three months, and the symptoms of an even smaller group may persist for six months or longer. To be sure that we were describing all potentially relevant care for every individual, we selected an observation period of six months, though not all care observed during this time period was necessarily associated with the mTBI.

To understand patterns of care over the six-month period, we defined several time segments of treatment following the mTBI diagnosis, including treatment received within the first 24 hours and every week thereafter, to see when a patient received care. We examined the timing of any type of care (we did not identify specific diagnoses or procedures), subsequent care associated with an mTBI diagnosis (based on personal history of TBI diagnosis, V15.52), care for co-occurring symptoms, and care for behavioral health diagnoses.

We also examined the characteristics and health care utilization of a subset of the 2012 mTBI cohort who were observed to have persistent care needs—that is, the population that received ongoing mTBI-related care for longer than three months after the mTBI diagnosis. We defined those with *persistent mTBI care needs* as service members with a new mTBI diagnosis who received mTBI-related care for 90 days or more. We defined *mTBI-related care* as any health care encounter for a service member with an associated personal history of TBI diagnostic code (V15.52). This was likely a conservative estimate of the population with persistent mTBI care needs, as it is unclear how consistent the use of this secondary code is across the MHS.[6]

To identify potential risk factors for needing persistent care, we calculated the relative risk for demographic and service history characteristics. Relative risk indicates the strength of association between a characteristic and an outcome in cohort studies such as this one. In our analysis, we compared one specific subgroup in a category (for example, "black, non-Hispanic" within "race") to all other subgroups in that category combined (all other races combined). This allowed us to identify which personal and service characteristics were risk factors for developing persistent problems. We adjusted the relative risk for potential confounding variables using a multivariate regression model. These confounding variables included gender, age, race, marital status, TRICARE region, history of TBI, service branch, cumulative months of deployment, years of service, and history of deployment.

---

[6] Relying on code V15.52 may underestimate the total number of service members who received care related to an mTBI. We show some relationships to other mTBI sequelae–type codes in Appendix B. For example, 58 percent of service members in our data with the diagnostic code for PCS also had a V15.52 diagnostic. Likewise, 94 percent of service members in our data with diagnostic codes for late effects from an intracranial injury or skull fracture had a V15.52 diagnostic code.

To more clearly identify the population with ongoing care needs, we also examined the size and characteristics of the population of service members who received treatment for PCS in 2012. PCS is clinically defined by a cluster of physical symptoms that persist for three months or more after a concussion. We considered this group separately from the cohort with a new mTBI; while the PCS group received care in 2012 for common or occasional symptoms and conditions that can co-occur with mTBI, that care may have been associated with an older mTBI rather than a new mTBI. We also identified all service members who had at least one health care encounter with an ICD-9 diagnosis code for PCS (310.2) in 2012 (n = 4,443).

Service Member and Clinical Care Variables

We describe the *demographic and service history characteristics* of the population of service members who received a diagnosis for a new mTBI in 2012 (in Chapter Three), as well as for the population of service members with a PCS diagnosis in 2012 (in Chapter Eight). For each of these groups, we report sex, age, race/ethnicity, marital status, TRICARE region, branch of service, and rank as categorical variables. We also report years of service and whether the service member had a history of deployment.[7] We used DMDC data to identify whether a service member had deployed since 2001, either to a location with a designated combat zone or area of operation or in direct support of these deployments. Those who had deployed since 2001 were characterized as having a *history of deployment* relative to those who had not. For characteristics that change over time (e.g., age), we report the value of the characteristic at the time of the first visit for the new mTBI.

To characterize an individual's *history of TBI*, we identified service members who had received a diagnosis for a new TBI (of any severity) in the years preceding the mTBI diagnosis in 2012. To do so, we applied the same clean-period criteria—six months with no visits with a TBI diagnosis followed by a visit with a TBI diagnosis—for all health care encounters between 2008 and 2011. We categorized service members as having a history of TBI if they were in the 2012 mTBI cohort and received a diagnosis for at least one TBI between 2008 and 2011.

Co-Occurring Diagnoses

We used two methods to identify relevant diagnoses that commonly or occasionally co-occur with mTBI. First, we reviewed the mTBI literature to develop a list of symptoms and co-occurring conditions (Borgaro et al., 2003; Lundin et al., 2006; Vaishnavi, Rao, and Fann, 2009). Second, we examined the frequency of all ICD-9 codes associated with health care encounters in the six months following the first (diagnosis) visit for mTBI in our study population. We report on a subset of co-occurring conditions that are either commonly reported in the literature or frequently experienced by the mTBI cohort. Additional detail about the ICD-9 codes used to define these conditions can be found in Appendix D.

- *Behavioral health conditions:* adjustment disorders, PTSD, other anxiety disorders (e.g., anxiety disorder not otherwise specified, panic disorder, obsessive compulsive disorder

---

[7] Our deployment data included service members who were physically located within a designated combat zone or area of operation or who were specifically identified by their service as directly supporting Operation Enduring Freedom or Operation Iraqi Freedom deployments. These data were extracted from DMDC's Contingency Tracking System.

[OCD], generalized anxiety disorder), depression (major depressive disorder, dysthymia), acute stress disorders, bipolar disorder, delirium or dementia, attention deficit or attention deficit and hyperactivity disorder (ADD/ADHD), alcohol abuse or dependence, and drug abuse or dependence.

- *Symptoms commonly or occasionally co-occurring with mTBI:* headache, other chronic pain, sleep disorders, irritability, memory loss, dizziness/vertigo, hearing problems, PCS, syncope and collapse, cognitive problems, skin sensation disturbances, alteration in mental status, gait and coordination problems, vision problems, communication disorders, and smell and taste disturbances.

Treatment Source and Setting

We characterized the treatment settings where service members in the mTBI cohort received care. We distinguished between *direct care*, which is care received at MTFs, and *purchased care*, which is care received in the community and paid for by TRICARE. In addition, we categorized the *setting of care*, the physical locations where service members in the mTBI cohort received care. For treatment received in the direct and purchased care systems, we identified whether the setting was a primary care clinic, emergency department, behavioral health specialty clinic, neurology clinic, inpatient facility, or other location.[8] Additional detail about how these settings were defined is available in Appendix D.

Diagnostic Assessments, Therapies, and Medications

While the predominant treatments for mTBI are time and patient education, some individuals with mTBI diagnoses receive additional treatment for certain symptoms or co-occurring conditions. We identified diagnostic assessments, therapies, and medications relevant to the treatment of symptoms and conditions that can co-occur with mTBI, using an approach similar to that described for co-occurring diagnoses. First, we reviewed DoD/VA clinical practice guidelines for the treatment of mTBI (VA and DoD, 2009) and clinical guidance for the treatment of related symptoms (e.g., headache; see DVBIC, 2009, 2013, and DCoE, 2012). From these records, we developed a list of relevant assessments, therapies, and medications. In addition, we reviewed the literature on the treatment of mTBI and consulted with our expert advisory group to identify additional treatments to include. Finally, we examined the frequency of all procedure codes (Current Procedural Terminology, or CPT, codes) associated with health care visits made by the cohort population in the six months following the diagnostic visit. Thus, we report on a subset of diagnostic assessments, therapies, and medications that were recommended by clinical practice guidelines or the expert advisory group, commonly reported in the literature, or received by the mTBI cohort. Additional detail about the CPT codes used to define these treatments is available in Appendix D.

---

[8] While we were able to identify whether service members in the mTBI cohort received care through the Veterans Health Administration (VHA), fewer than 1 percent of all health care encounters fell into this category and are therefore not reported separately.

CHAPTER THREE

How Many Service Members Receive Treatment for mTBI?

In this chapter, we describe the number of nondeployed active-duty service members who received treatment through the MHS for common or occasional symptoms and conditions that can co-occur with mTBI, comparing our estimates with previously reported estimates. We also identify the number of service members with a new diagnosis of mTBI in 2012.[1]

Number of Nondeployed Active-Duty Service Members with mTBI, 2008–2013

To assess changes in the number of service members receiving treatment for common or occasional symptoms and conditions that can co-occur with mTBI over time, we first examined the number of nondeployed active-duty service members who received an mTBI diagnosis between 2008 and 2013, regardless of whether it was a new diagnosis. Figure 3.1 shows that the number of active-component personnel each year who had a health care encounter, for any reason, during which they received an mTBI diagnosis was relatively steady between 2009 and 2012, ranging from 20,600 to 21,800. Slightly fewer service members received care for an mTBI diagnosis in 2008, and, because our data were complete only through June 2013, we undercount the number of nondeployed active-duty service members with an mTBI diagnosis in 2013.

Comparing the RAND Estimate to DoD Estimates

The rest of the analyses in this report focus on the population of nondeployed active-duty service members who received treatment following a documented ICD-9 code of mTBI in 2012. To understand whether and how our application of the case definition for mTBI in these data affected estimates of the size of the mTBI population, we compared our estimate of the number of service members with mTBI in 2012 to estimates published by DoD (DVBIC, 2014a; based on data from the Defense Medical Surveillance System and the Theater Medical Data Store). Table 3.1 presents the DoD estimates for 2012 and compares them with the data from this study. It is important to note that most DoD estimates include both active- and reserve-component service members. Although reserve-component personnel are a critical part of the DoD community, we do not include them in our analyses because it is possible that a portion of their health care visits are not captured in TRICARE data. While eligible

---

[1] Recall that a new mTBI diagnosis is defined as a diagnosis of mTBI following a six-month clean period in which the service member did not receive any treatment for a TBI diagnosis (of any severity).

Figure 3.1
Number of Nondeployed Active-Duty Service Members Who Received an mTBI Diagnosis, 2008–2013

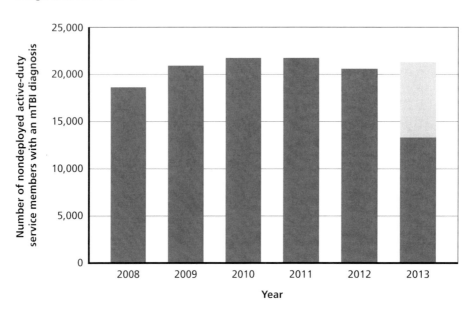

NOTES: TRICARE encounter data were extracted on or around October 24, 2013. Direct care data are considered complete within 90 days of an encounter; purchased care data are complete within 120 days. Therefore, the data extract used for this study contained complete direct and purchased care data through the end of June 2013. We extrapolated through the end of the calendar year to generate an estimate of 21,212 mTBI cases in 2013.
RAND RR844-3.1

for TRICARE during periods of activation (and for six months after returning from a deployment), these service members may retain some form of private insurance, and this care would not be included in our data. It is also important to note that our estimates do not include mTBI diagnoses received in theater.

To ensure that our comparison was based on similar populations, we considered the active-duty portion of the DoD estimate, which is most comparable to our data, separately from the DoD total force estimate, which includes National Guard and reserve personnel (see Table 3.1). These results suggest that our estimates are similar to those reported by DoD.

Nondeployed Active-Duty Service Members with a mTBI New Diagnosis in 2012

After applying the clean period and other exclusions noted in Chapter Two, we identified 16,378 nondeployed active-duty service members with a new mTBI diagnosis in 2012. As expected, the number of service members who received treatment for a new mTBI diagnosis (n = 16,378) was smaller than the number who received treatment for any mTBI diagnosis (n = 20,638).

Because we could not observe injuries and diagnoses that occurred in theater, and because service members receive thorough health assessments when they return from a deployment, we examined the frequency of mTBI diagnoses shortly after that period. Among those who received treatment for a new mTBI diagnosis in 2012, 9 percent were diagnosed within

Table 3.1
Comparing DoD mTBI Estimates to mTBI Estimates Using Project Data

mTBI Diagnoses	DoD Estimates		Project Data
	2012 Active Duty	2012 Total	
Overall	21,319	26,127	20,638
Service			
Army	12,506	16,178	10,980
Navy	2,704	2,957	2,813
Air Force	2,702	3,285	3,160
Marine Corps	3,407	3,707	3,134

SOURCE: DVBIC, 2014c.

NOTE: Service numbers in the "Project Data" column do not sum due to missing data.

30 days of returning from a deployment. While this finding suggests that some service members in the 2012 mTBI cohort sustained an injury in theater and were diagnosed during the post-deployment health assessment, it also suggests that many of the mTBIs observed in this data were not deployment-related.

Conclusions

In this chapter, we reported the number of nondeployed active-duty service members diagnosed with an mTBI over time, regardless of whether it was a new diagnosis, as well the number of service members who had a new diagnosis of mTBI in 2012.

Between 2008 and 2009, the number of service members with an mTBI diagnosis increased (from approximately 18,700 to nearly 22,000), after which the number of diagnosed service members remained roughly steady through 2012. Once we imposed a six-month clean period with no TBI diagnosis, we identified 16,378 active-component service members who received a new diagnosis of mTBI in 2012. Throughout the rest of the report, we focus on this population of nondeployed active-duty service members who received a diagnosis for a new mTBI in 2012.

CHAPTER FOUR

What Are the Characteristics of Nondeployed Active-Duty Service Members Who Receive Treatment for an mTBI Through the MHS?

In this chapter, we describe the characteristics of the cohort of nondeployed active-duty service members diagnosed with a new mTBI in 2012. Specifically, we describe their demographic and service history characteristics and co-occurring conditions for which they received treatment during the six months following their mTBI diagnosis. We also examine differences in these characteristics by service and whether the service members had been treated for a previous TBI.

Demographic Characteristics of 2012 mTBI Cohort

As Table 4.1 shows, nondeployed active-duty service members in the 2012 mTBI cohort tended to be male (87 percent); young (e.g., 48 percent were 18–24; 38 percent were 25–34); white, non-Hispanic (65 percent); and married (56 percent). Ten percent had a history of TBI (a previous TBI observed in our data between 2008 and 2011). Table 4.1 also includes data on the demographic characteristics of the entire active-component population in 2012 (DoD, 2013). The sex, race, and marital status of the 2012 mTBI cohort and the overall population of service members were very similar. However, the 2012 mTBI cohort tended to be younger than the population as a whole, with 48 percent of the cohort in the 18–24 age range, compared with 43 percent in the overall service member population.[1]

Next, we describe the demographic characteristics of the 2012 mTBI cohort by service branch. All differences by service were statistically significant (p < 0.0001). As Table 4.2 shows, Army personnel made up the majority of new mTBI cases in 2012. The other three services were roughly evenly divided at 13–16 percent of all new mTBI diagnoses in 2012. While service members with mTBI were predominantly male across service branches, the Air Force had the highest percentage of women (20 percent), and the Marine Corps had the lowest (8 percent). Among all service branches, service members with mTBI tended to be young. However, in the Marine Corps, those with mTBI were younger than those in the other service branches, with 64 percent aged 18–24, compared with 43–51 percent in the other services. Those with mTBI were mostly white, non-Hispanic across all services, but Navy personnel were more likely than other service members to be nonwhite. Most Army personnel with mTBI were married (63 percent), compared with fewer than 50 percent in the other services. They were also the most likely to have a history of TBI, while Navy personnel were the least likely (12.2 percent and 5.4 percent, respectively).

---

[1] The age categories are not identical but vary only slightly.

Table 4.1
Demographic Characteristics of the 2012 mTBI Cohort

Demographic Characteristic	Number of Nondeployed Active-Duty Service Members	% of 2012 mTBI Cohort (n = 16,378)	% of All Service Members in 2012 (n = 1,388,028)
Sex			
Female	2,176	13.3	14.6
Male	14,202	86.7	85.4
Age (age at diagnosis for cohort population)			
18–24	7,861	48.0	42.7 (25 or younger)
25–34	6,157	37.6	37.7 (26–35)
35–44	2,031	12.4	19.7 (36+)
45 and over	329	2.0	
Race/ethnicity			
American Indian/Alaskan Native	297	1.8	1.5
Asian or Pacific Islander	630	3.8	3.7
Black, non-Hispanic	2,319	14.2	16.8
White, non-Hispanic	10,699	65.3	69.7
Hispanic	1,843	11.3	(not reported)
Other/unknown	590	3.6	8.3
Marital status			
Married	9,149	55.9	56.1
Never married	6,444	39.3	39.3
Divorced, separated, or widowed	778	4.8	4.6
Region			
TRICARE North	4,421	27.0	27.9
TRICARE South	3,335	20.4	26.6
TRICARE West	6,930	42.3	32.5
TRICARE Overseas	1,539	9.4	12.5
Unknown	153	0.9	—
TBI history, 2008–2011	1,611	9.8	—

SOURCE: Percentages of all service members in 2012 from DoD, 2013.

NOTE: Numbers may not sum due to missing data.

Table 4.2
Demographic Characteristics of the 2012 mTBI Cohort, by Service

Demographic Characteristic	% in Service Branch (number and % of mTBI Cohort			
	Army (n = 8,791, 54%)	Navy (n = 2,191, 13%)	Air Force (2,686, 16%)	Marine Corps (n = 2,248, 14%)
Sex				
Female	11.1	17.0	20.2	8.0
Male	88.9	83.0	79.8	92.0
Age at diagnosis				
18–24	42.8	50.1	51.2	64.3
25–34	41.0	35.3	35.6	28.6
35–44	14.0	12.3	11.5	6.6
45–64	2.2	2.3	1.7	0.4
65 and over	0.0	0.0	0.0	0.0
Race/ethnicity				
American Indian/Alaskan Native	1.1	5.5	1.0	1.6
Asian or Pacific Islander	4.1	4.8	3.3	3.2
Black, non-Hispanic	15.7	15.1	13.2	10.4
White, non-Hispanic	65.9	48.2	71.8	71.6
Hispanic	12.0	15.7	4.4	12.1
Other/unknown	1.2	10.7	6.3	1.1
Marital status				
Married	63.2	46.2	48.3	46.4
Never married	31.6	51.1	45.6	50.3
Divorced, separated, or widowed	5.1	2.5	6.0	3.4
Region				
TRICARE North	24.0	37.6	13.3	40.7
TRICARE South	21.8	18.2	28.8	5.7
TRICARE West	43.2	36.7	45.7	43.5
TRICARE Overseas	9.8	7.5	11.4	8.8
Unknown	1.1	0.0	0.9	1.3
TBI history, 2008–2011	12.2	5.4	7.0	8.5

NOTES: N = 16,378. All differences are significant at $p < 0.001$. Service numbers and percentages do not sum due to missing data on 462 service members.

Service Characteristics of 2012 mTBI Cohort

Table 4.3 describes the service characteristics of the 2012 mTBI cohort, both overall and by service branch. (All differences by service branch were statistically significant, p < 0.0001.) Half of all nondeployed active-duty service members with a new mTBI diagnosis in 2012 were junior enlisted at the time of diagnosis, though a larger proportion of marines were junior-ranked (two-thirds were E1–E4) compared with those from the other services (Cameron et al., 2012). On average, nondeployed active-duty service members with a new mTBI had completed six years of service. The results for both the rank and years of service are consistent with the age composition of these populations, as shown in Table 4.3.

Two-thirds of the 2012 mTBI cohort had a history of deployment. On average, those with a history of deployment had been deployed for 16 cumulative months prior to their mTBI diagnosis. These numbers vary by service, with Army personnel considerably more likely to have been deployed (79 percent), and for seven to nine months longer, than personnel from the other service branches.

Co-Occurring Diagnoses

To this point, we have considered only mTBI diagnoses, but most treatment for TBI is symptom-based. Common symptoms associated with mTBI include headache, sleep dysfunction, dizziness, and balance disorders (DCoE and DVBIC, 2010). In addition, mTBI is frequently co-occurring with behavioral health conditions, such as depression and PTSD (Carlson et al., 2011; Hoge, McGurk, et al., 2008).

Table 4.3
Service Characteristics of the 2012 mTBI Cohort, Overall and by Service

Service Characteristic	% Overall (n = 16,378)	% in Service Branch			
		Army (n = 8,791)	Navy (n = 2,191)	Air Force (n = 2,686)	Marine Corps (n = 2,248)
Rank at diagnosis					
E1–E4	53.6	52.7	50.2	50.7	65.7
E5–E9	34.8	36.9	35.1	33.2	29.0
O1–O3	6.1	6.1	6.0	7.6	3.6
O4–O6	2.7	2.3	3.5	3.7	1.6
Other/unknown	2.7	2.0	5.3	4.8	0.0
Years of service (mean)	6.2	6.3	6.5	6.4	5.1
Deployment history					
Ever deployed (2001–diagnosis)	66.3	79.2	54.1	50.7	58.1
Cumulative months deployed (prior to diagnosis), among those ever deployed	15.8	18.8	9.9	9.5	11.5

NOTES: N = 16,378. All differences by service are statistically significant at p < 0.0001. Service numbers do not sum due to missing data on 462 service members.

We had two analytic motivations for understanding treatment received by the 2012 mTBI cohort for diagnoses other than mTBI. Most importantly, diagnostic coding guidance recommends that an mTBI diagnosis be recorded only during the first visit, so, to describe follow-up care, we had to identify the care received for diagnoses that were potentially associated with the mTBI. Second, to put into context the frequency, intensity, and duration of care, it was important to determine the complexity of the population's health care needs. Those with multiple conditions or a range of co-occurring symptoms may need more intense or different types of treatment; therefore, a description of the other conditions we observed helped frame our interpretation of the care that was delivered.

Treatment for Co-Occurring Behavioral Health Conditions

Table 4.4 shows the proportion of the 2012 mTBI cohort that received any treatment for selected behavioral health conditions in the six months following the initial mTBI diagnosis. We expected that this population would have high rates of behavioral health problems, as this has been demonstrated in previous studies (Hoge, McGurk, et al., 2008; Lew, Poole, et al., 2007), though the relationship between mTBI and behavioral health problems may not be causal (Wilk et al., 2012). Treatment for adjustment disorders (16 percent) and anxiety disorders (14 percent) was the most common, followed by treatment for depression, alcohol abuse and dependence, and PTSD. The remainder of the conditions had a much lower rate of co-occurrence (approximately 3 percent or less).

We examined the proportion of the mTBI cohort that received treatment for behavioral health conditions both before and after the mTBI diagnosis, indicating ongoing treatment for these conditions. We then compared this number to the number who received treatment only after the mTBI diagnosis (see Figure 4.1). For most of the behavioral health conditions we

Table 4.4
Treatment for Behavioral Health Conditions in the Six
Months After mTBI Diagnosis

Behavioral Health Condition	% of 2012 mTBI Cohort
Adjustment disorders	16.0
Anxiety disorders	14.4
Depression	12.4
Alcohol abuse/dependence	11.2
PTSD	11.0
ADD/ADHD	2.7
Delirium/dementia	2.4
Drug abuse/dependence	2.1
Acute stress disorders	1.4
Bipolar disorder	0.8

NOTES: N = 16,378. Anxiety disorders include generalized anxiety disorder, OCD, anxiety not otherwise specified, and panic disorder. Depression includes major depressive disorder and dysthymia.

Figure 4.1
Treatment for Behavioral Health Conditions in the Six Months Before and After mTBI Diagnosis

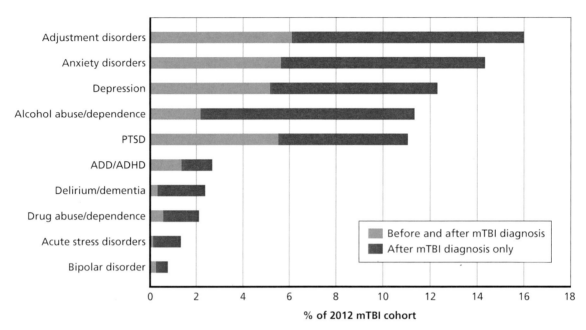

NOTES: Anxiety disorders include generalized anxiety disorder, OCD, anxiety not otherwise specified, and panic disorder. Depression includes major depressive disorder and dysthymia.
RAND RR844-4.1

examined, about 30–50 percent of those who received treatment in the six months after the mTBI diagnosis also received treatment in the six months prior to the mTBI diagnosis. Notably, only 20 percent of those who received treatment for alcohol abuse or dependence in the six months after the mTBI diagnosis had received alcohol treatment in the six months before the mTBI diagnosis. Previous work has suggested that substance abuse is a risk factor for mTBI, perhaps related to an increased risk of motor vehicle accidents or falls. Further, service members with an mTBI may be at increased risk for substance abuse following the injury, though existing findings on this question are mixed (Miller et al., 2013).

There are several possible explanations for this pattern of pre- and post-mTBI health care use for behavioral health conditions more broadly. Behavioral health conditions could have developed as a consequence of an mTBI or as a psychiatric response to the same event in which the service member was injured. Alternatively, preexisting behavioral health conditions could have been identified because of the patient's contact with the health care system.

Differences in the Receipt of Treatment for Co-Occurring Behavioral Health Conditions, by TBI History

Treatment for all behavioral health diagnoses was more common among those with a history of TBI (of any severity), with service members with a previous TBI twice as likely to be diagnosed as those with no history of TBI (Figure 4.2). Most differences by TBI history were statistically significant (p < 0.0001), though there was no difference by TBI history in the rates of treatment for alcohol abuse/dependence or ADD/ADHD. The finding that those with a TBI history were generally more likely to receive treatment for a co-occurring behavioral health condition may be expected, as previous research has found that repeated TBIs increase the risk

Figure 4.2
Treatment for Behavioral Health Conditions in the Six Months After mTBI Diagnosis, by TBI History

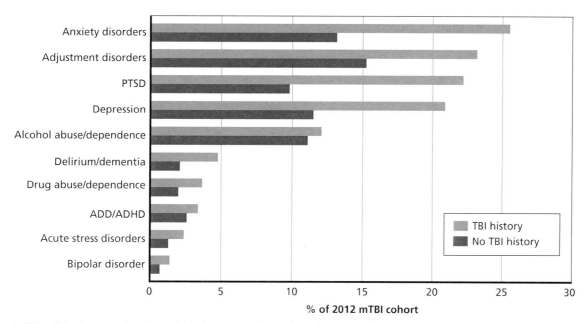

NOTE: With the exception of alcohol abuse/dependence (p-value = 0.218) and ADD/ADHD (p-value = 0.0758) treatment, all treatment differences were statistically significant at p < 0.0001.
RAND RR844-4.2

of certain behavioral health conditions (Anstey et al., 2004; Schneiderman, Braver, and Kang, 2008) and anxiety.

Individuals with mTBI may receive treatment for more than one co-occurring behavioral health condition. As a starting point to illustrate how behavioral health conditions may co-occur within the mTBI cohort, Table 4.5 shows the frequency of each behavioral health condition (columns) conditional on experiencing other conditions (rows). So, for example, 38 percent of those with adjustment disorders also experience anxiety disorder. In contrast, 42 percent of those with anxiety disorders also experience adjustment disorders. Looking down the columns, it is easy to see that the rates of some conditions are relatively independent of other conditions. Other conditions show strong dependencies, however. For example, anxiety disorders (generalized anxiety disorder, OCD, anxiety not otherwise specified, and panic disorder) were much more common among those experiencing PTSD than among those with alcohol use and dependence problems. The table indicates that behavioral health conditions often co-occurred and may have formed clusters of symptoms within this cohort.

Treatment for Symptoms and Conditions Commonly or Occasionally Associated with mTBI in the Six Months Following a New mTBI Diagnosis

Next, we describe the proportion of the 2012 mTBI cohort that received treatment for nonbehavioral health conditions and symptoms in the six months following the new mTBI diagnosis (Table 4.6). Treatment for non-headache pain conditions (57 percent) and headache (40 percent) was most common.[2] Treatment for sleep disorders was also common, with one-quarter of

---

[2] Non-headache pain and other symptoms and conditions may be associated with other causes, such as extracranial trauma, that may co-occur with mTBI.

Table 4.5
Co-Occurrence of Treatment for Behavioral Health Conditions in the Six Months After mTBI Diagnosis

Diagnosis	Incidence in mTBI Cohort (n)	% of 2012 mTBI Cohort with Co-Occurring Diagnosis									
		Adjustment Disorders	Anxiety Disorders	Depression	Alcohol Abuse/ Dependence	PTSD	Delirium/ Dementia	ADD/ADHD	Drug Abuse/ Dependence	Acute Stress Disorders	Bipolar Disorder
Adjustment disorders	2,617	100.0	38.4	35.9	17.2	28.8	5.0	6.6	6.2	4.8	2.3
Anxiety disorders	2,361	42.5	100.0	44.1	17.9	41.0	6.7	8.2	7.3	4.6	3.5
Depression	2,037	46.1	51.2	100.0	23.1	45.9	7.1	9.1	8.0	4.4	4.3
Alcohol abuse/ dependence	1,832	24.6	23.0	25.7	100.0	20.6	3.5	4.1	11.0	2.7	2.5
PTSD	1,800	41.8	53.7	51.9	20.9	100.0	8.6	8.0	7.9	5.8	4.2
Delirium/ dementia	394	33.0	40.4	36.5	16.2	39.3	100.0	6.6	5.3	4.6	2.8
ADD/ADHD	438	39.5	44.3	42.2	17.1	32.9	5.9	100.0	8.4	3.0	5.7
Drug abuse/ dependence	347	46.7	49.9	47.0	57.9	40.9	6.1	10.7	100.0	4.6	8.1
Acute stress disorders	234	53.4	46.2	38.0	20.9	44.9	7.7	5.6	6.8	100.0	4.3
Bipolar disorder	128	46.9	64.8	68.0	35.2	58.6	8.6	19.5	21.9	7.8	100.0

NOTES: Anxiety disorders include generalized anxiety disorder, OCD, anxiety not otherwise specified, and panic disorder. Depression includes major depressive disorder and dysthymia.

Table 4.6
Treatment for Symptoms and Conditions Commonly or Occasionally Associated with mTBI in the Six Months After mTBI Diagnosis

Diagnosis	% of 2012 mTBI Cohort
Non-headache pain condition	57.0
Headache	39.7
Sleep disorders and symptoms	25.6
Memory loss	15.6
Dizziness/vertigo	11.0
Hearing problems	9.0
PCS	6.6
Irritability	5.9
Syncope and collapse	5.5
Cognitive problems	5.2
Skin sensation disturbances	3.9
Alteration in mental status	3.8
Gait and coordination problems	3.8
Vision problems	2.7
Communication disorders	1.4
Smell and taste disturbances	0.2

NOTE: N = 16,378.

the 2012 mTBI cohort receiving treatment for a sleep disorder. Small proportions of the 2012 mTBI cohort received treatment for other conditions and symptoms. This is consistent with the findings of studies of civilian populations, which have found that pain conditions, head aches, and sleep disorders are common in the months after an mTBI (Nicholson, 2000; Perlis, Artiola, and Giles, 1997; Vanderploeg, Belanger, and Curtiss, 2009).

Since treatment for these symptoms and conditions may be unrelated to the mTBI, we examined the proportion of the mTBI cohort that received treatment for these symptoms and conditions in the six months before and after the mTBI diagnosis, suggesting ongoing treatment, compared with those who received treatment only in the six months after the mTBI diagnosis (Figure 4.3). For most of the symptoms and conditions we examined, a relatively low proportion of the cohort received treatment in the six months before the mTBI diagnosis. About half of those who received treatment for non-headache pain in the six months after the mTBI diagnosis also received treatment for non-headache pain in the six months prior to the mTBI diagnosis.

As illustrated in Figure 4.4, those with a prior TBI were generally more likely than those without a history of TBI to receive treatment for each condition. Treatment for non-headache pain conditions was common in both groups, with 68 percent of those with a previ-

Figure 4.3
Treatment for Symptoms and Conditions Commonly or Occasionally Associated with mTBI in the Six Months Before and After mTBI Diagnosis

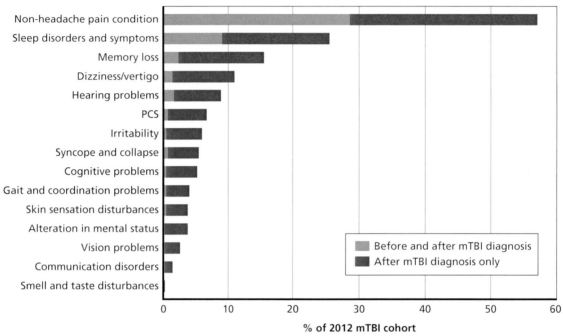

ous TBI and 56 percent of those without a history of TBI receiving treatment for this condition (statistically significant difference at p < 0.001). Service members with a previous TBI were much more likely to have received treatment for a sleep disorder (40 percent) and memory loss (27 percent) compared with those without a history of TBI (24 and 15 percent, respectively; p < 0.0001 for both).

Since it is common to experience multiple symptoms in the aftermath of an mTBI, we explored clusters of symptoms and conditions in our cohort. Table 4.7 shows the frequency of each condition or symptom (columns) conditional on experiencing other conditions or symptoms (rows). Looking down the columns, it is clear that some conditions and symptoms (e.g., non-headache pain) are relatively independent of other conditions or symptoms. Other conditions and symptoms show strong associations, however. For example, sleep disorders and symptoms were much more common among those experiencing memory loss, irritability, and cognitive problems than among those experiencing pain, PCS, syncope and collapse, or an alteration in mental status.

Conclusions

In this chapter, we described the demographic and service characteristics of nondeployed active-duty service members who received a diagnosis for a new mTBI in 2012. They tended to be young, male, junior enlisted, and white, non-Hispanic. Just more than half of the cohort was composed of Army personnel, and the remainder was evenly split across the other three

Figure 4.4
Treatment for Symptoms and Conditions Commonly or Occasionally Associated with mTBI in the Six Months After mTBI Diagnosis, by TBI History

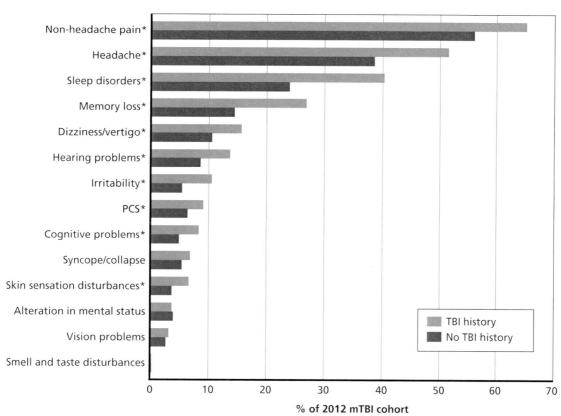

*Statistically significant difference at p < 0.0001.

RAND RR844-4.4

services. Two-thirds of the cohort had deployment experience at the time of diagnosis, and, on average, these service members had deployed for 16 months.

We also considered treatment for conditions and symptoms in the six months before and after an mTBI diagnosis. While 5–10 percent of the cohort received treatment for behavioral health conditions, including anxiety disorders, adjustment disorders, PTSD, depression, and alcohol abuse/dependence, in the six months after mTBI diagnoses, some service members were receiving care for these conditions prior to their mTBI diagnosis. Thus, the relationship between mTBI and other behavioral health conditions, as presented here, should not be interpreted as causal but, rather, co-occurring. While the events and injuries may indeed be causal in a medical sense, the data do not allow us to determine causality. Service members with a history of TBI (of any severity) prior to 2012 were much more likely to receive treatment for these behavioral health conditions.

Finally, we analyzed the rate of co-occurrence of nonbehavioral health conditions and symptoms. Non-headache pain, headaches, and sleep disorders were the most common conditions that were treated during the six months following the diagnosis of mTBI. Service members with a history of TBI were more likely to be treated for co-occurring symptoms and conditions.

Table 4.7
Co-Occurrence of Treatment for Symptoms and Conditions Commonly or Occasionally Associated with mTBI in the Six Months After mTBI Diagnosis

Diagnosis	Incidence in mTBI Cohort (n)	% of 2012 mTBI Cohort with Co-Occurring Diagnosis							
		Non-Headache Pain Condition	Headache	Sleep Disorders and Symptoms	Memory Loss	Dizziness/ Vertigo	Hearing Problems	PCS	Irritability
Non-headache pain condition	9,335	100.0	47.3	33.4	20.3	13.8	11.8	7.6	7.3
Headache	6,508	67.9	100.0	42.0	29.8	20.7	14.9	11.4	10.8
Sleep disorders and symptoms	4,200	74.2	65.1	100.0	42.8	22.0	21.5	9.6	18.0
Memory loss	2,562	74.1	75.6	70.1	100.0	30.5	27.5	13.3	23.8
Dizziness/vertigo	1,807	71.2	74.4	51.0	43.3	100.0	24.0	16.0	15.4
Hearing problems	1,468	74.7	66.1	61.6	48.0	29.5	100.0	11.4	18.3
PCS	1,083	65.7	68.3	37.4	31.6	26.8	15.4	100.0	5.9
Irritability	969	70.4	72.2	78.1	63.1	28.8	27.7	6.6	100.0
Syncope and collapse	902	63.0	48.4	29.7	14.6	25.6	8.4	9.4	5.0
Cognitive problems	852	78.2	75.7	70.2	71.6	34.5	29.0	17.3	20.5
Skin sensation disturbances	645	88.7	58.1	44.5	30.7	24.2	19.2	11.6	9.0
Alteration in mental status	630	71.7	46.0	29.2	21.9	16.2	9.7	11.1	4.3
Gait and coordination problems	687	86.2	65.1	65.4	60.3	43.1	32.8	18.3	15.6
Vision problems	441	68.3	58.5	43.5	39.2	26.8	17.9	12.9	11.6
Communication disorders	230	82.2	64.3	56.5	55.2	29.6	37.0	23.0	12.2
Smell and taste disturbances	29	79.3	75.9	55.2	58.6	37.9	20.7	24.1	13.8

Table 4.7— Continued

Diagnosis	% of 2012 mTBI Cohort with Co-Occurring Diagnosis							
	Syncope and Collapse	Cognitive Problems	Skin Sensation Disturbances	Alteration in Mental Status	Gait and Coordination Problems	Vision Problems	Communication Disorders	Smell and Taste Disturbances
Non-headache pain condition	6.1	7.1	6.1	4.8	6.3	3.2	2.0	0.2
Headache	6.7	9.9	5.8	4.5	6.9	4.0	2.3	0.3
Sleep disorders and symptoms	6.4	14.2	6.8	4.4	10.7	4.6	3.1	0.4
Memory loss	5.2	23.8	7.7	5.4	16.2	6.8	5.0	0.7
Dizziness/vertigo	12.8	16.3	8.6	5.6	16.4	6.5	3.8	0.6
Hearing problems	5.2	16.8	8.4	4.2	15.3	5.4	5.8	0.4
PCS	7.8	13.6	6.9	6.5	11.6	5.3	4.9	0.6
Irritability	4.6	18.1	6.0	2.8	11.0	5.3	2.9	0.4
Syncope and collapse	100.0	4.4	7.8	14.1	4.8	3.2	1.7	0.6
Cognitive problems	4.7	100.0	7.7	5.9	21.1	9.2	9.6	0.6
Skin sensation disturbances	10.9	10.2	100.0	6.7	13.5	5.9	3.7	0.5
Alteration in mental status	20.2	7.9	6.8	100.0	11.1	3.7	5.1	0.8
Gait and coordination problems	6.3	26.2	12.7	10.2	100.0	8.2	8.4	1.3
Vision problems	6.6	17.7	8.6	5.2	12.7	100.0	5.0	0.2
Communication disorders	6.5	35.7	10.4	13.9	25.2	9.6	100.0	0.9
Smell and taste disturbances	17.2	17.2	10.3	17.2	31.0	3.4	6.9	100.0

CHAPTER FIVE

Where Do Nondeployed Active-Duty Service Members with mTBI Receive Care?

In this chapter, we describe the location of care for nondeployed active-duty service members diagnosed with a new mTBI in 2012, exploring both the treatment setting for the initial mTBI diagnosis and the first health care encounter after diagnosis.

Location of Initial mTBI Diagnosis

Figures 5.1, 5.2, and 5.3 show the care settings where nondeployed active-duty service members received their initial mTBI diagnosis in 2012. Among all service members, more than half (58 percent) received their initial mTBI diagnosis at an MTF in the direct care system. Most service members who were diagnosed at an MTF received their diagnosis in primary care settings (39 percent of all initial diagnoses in the direct care system) or emergency department (35 percent). In the purchased care system, the vast majority were diagnosed in the emergency department (80 percent of all initial purchased care diagnoses). Across the direct and purchased care systems, approximately half of all service members with an mTBI received their initial diagnosis in an emergency department. This finding may reflect the nature of these data, which did not include care delivered in theater. The high rates of mTBI diagnoses in the emergency department suggest that the injuries were the result of incidents that occurred in garrison.

Figure 5.1
Care Setting for mTBI Diagnosis

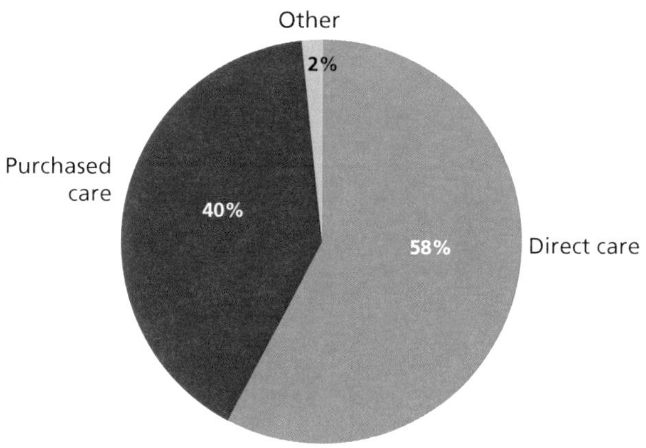

Figure 5.2
Location of mTBI Diagnosis in the Direct
Care System

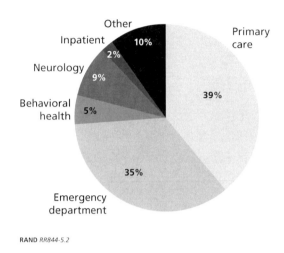

RAND RR844-5.2

Figure 5.3
Location of mTBI Diagnosis in the Purchased
Care System

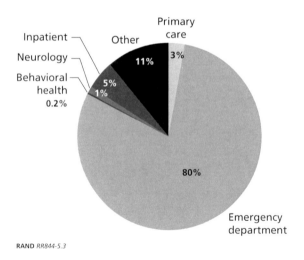

RAND RR844-5.3

Timing and Location of First Health Care Encounter After mTBI Diagnosis

Next, we consider when and where service members with a new mTBI in 2012 had their next health care encounter after their mTBI diagnosis.

Table 5.1 shows the average number of days between initial mTBI diagnosis and the next health care encounter. For the 2012 mTBI cohort, the next health care encounter occurred 16.7 days, on average, after the diagnosis. There is some variation by service, with Army and Air Force personnel having their next health care encounter approximately 15 days after diagnosis and Navy and Marine Corps personnel being seen approximately 20 days after diagnosis.

Table 5.1
Days Between mTBI Diagnosis and Next Health Care
Encounter, by Service, TBI History, and Deployment History

Population	Days Between Diagnosis and Next Health Care Encounter
Overall	16.7
Service	
Army	15.3
Navy	21.3
Air Force	14.9
Marine Corps	20.3
TBI history	
No previous TBI	11.2
Previous TBI	17.8
Deployment history	
Deployed	16.5
Never deployed	19.4

Figures 5.4, 5.5, and 5.6 show the locations where nondeployed active-duty service members had their next health care encounter after their mTBI diagnosis. The vast majority (87 percent) of subsequent visits occurred in the direct care setting, with nearly 40 percent of all visits in MTF primary care clinics. Purchased care made up only 11 percent of all next health care encounters after an mTBI diagnosis. A large percentage of service members had their next health care encounter in a location designated as "other," which most commonly included optometry, audiology, physical therapy, and radiology.

Figure 5.4
Location of Next Health Care Encounter After
mTBI Diagnosis

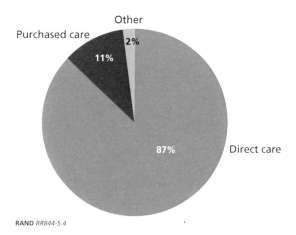

RAND RR844-5.4

Figure 5.5
Location of Next Health Care Encounter After mTBI
Diagnosis, Direct Care System

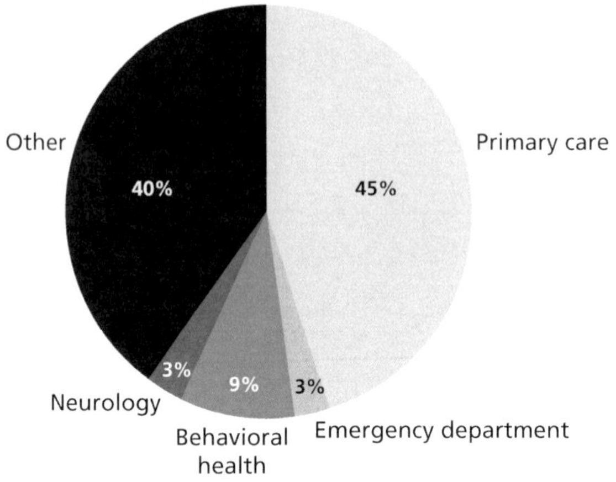

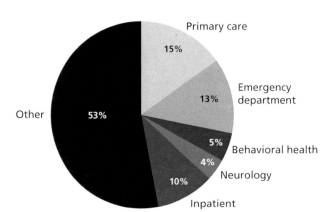

Other   40%

Primary care   45%

Neurology   3%

Behavioral health   9%

Emergency department   3%

NOTE: No members of the cohort had their next health care encounter in a direct care inpatient setting, so we excluded that category from this and subsequent figures.
RAND *RR844-5.5*

Figure 5.6
Location of Next Health Care Encounter, Purchased Care System

Primary care   15%

Emergency department   13%

Behavioral health   5%

Neurology   4%

Inpatient   10%

Other   53%

RAND *RR844-5.6*

Location of Care

Next, we considered care beyond the diagnosis visit and next health care encounter. Table 5.2 shows the percentage of service members in the 2012 mTBI cohort who received any care for any condition in various settings in the six months following diagnosis. Nearly all nondeployed active-duty service members received at least some of their care in a direct care setting, most of which was primary care. Forty percent of the mTBI cohort received treatment in an outpatient behavioral health specialty clinic (direct care), and one-third received treatment in a direct care emergency department setting. Twenty percent received care in an outpatient neurology clinic.

Table 5.2
Percentage of Service Members in the 2012 mTBI Cohort Who Received Any Care in the Six Months Following Diagnosis

Care Setting	% of 2012 mTBI Cohort
Direct care (any)	97.1
Primary care	81.9
Emergency department	35.2
Neurology	19.4
Behavioral health	41.1
Inpatient	6.6
Purchased care (any)	62.3

NOTE: N = 16,378.

In addition, nearly two-thirds of the cohort received at least some care through the purchased care network.

Conclusions

In 2012, approximately 60 percent of all service members with a new mTBI diagnosis received their diagnosis at an MTF, split somewhat evenly among primary care, emergency department, and all other locations. For the remaining 40 percent diagnosed in the purchased care network, the majority of diagnoses occurred in civilian emergency departments.

Most mTBI patients had another health care encounter approximately two weeks after their mTBI diagnosis, though Navy and Marine Corps personnel were seen closer to three weeks later. The vast majority (87 percent) had their next health care encounter in the direct care network, primarily in primary care settings.

For all care beyond the first health care encounter following the diagnosis visit, we reported the percentage of the cohort that received any care in a variety of settings. Almost all of those in the 2012 mTBI cohort had at least one health care encounter in the direct care setting, and 80 percent received care in a primary care clinic. Emergency departments and behavioral health clinics were other common locations for subsequent care, with 35–40 percent of the cohort receiving care in these settings. Two-thirds of the cohort received some care through the purchased care network.

CHAPTER SIX

What Are the Duration and Patterns of Health Care in the Six Months After an mTBI Diagnosis?

In this chapter, we present results from our analysis of health care received by nondeployed active-duty service members during the first six months following an mTBI diagnosis. First, we profile health care use in the six months following the mTBI diagnosis. Although the data did not allow us to attribute care subsequent to the mTBI diagnosis to mTBI treatment, we identified the amount of time service members received health care after an mTBI diagnosis and the types of diagnoses made during these visits. Second, we describe patterns of care for the 2012 cohort over the six months following the mTBI diagnosis. This allowed us to determine how certain types of care are being used over time and to compare the patterns we observed for one type of care with patterns for another.

Duration of Care in the 2012 mTBI Cohort

As previously discussed, DoD ICD-9 coding guidance for TBI recommends that a TBI diagnosis be reported during the initial visit only, and subsequent visits should be coded with a diagnosis for the primary symptom with a diagnostic code for a "personal history of TBI" (V15.52) to indicate that the treatment being provided is related to the TBI (DoD, 2010). However, personal history codes are used inconsistently in practice. Many providers fail to use them at all. Others use mTBI diagnoses repeatedly. Some use personal history codes during the second visit and later, though it is not clear when such codes should be dropped from records. Patterns of care among individual patients, furthermore, may make it difficult or impossible to use personal history codes properly, even among providers who follow DoD coding guidance. For example, many patients are seen in several care settings that do not have access to records from other settings. For this reason, an initial mTBI diagnosis may be repeated in a single patient's record each time he or she receives care in a new setting.

Because personal history codes are used inconsistently in practice, it is difficult to know whether treatment received subsequent to a TBI diagnosis is related to the TBI or whether care was provided for conditions unrelated to the TBI. This makes tracking patients over time difficult, and, therefore, it is a challenge to accurately describe an episode of care for mTBI.

To address this challenge, we sought to gain a better understanding of how long service members interact with the health care system after an mTBI diagnosis, on the premise that this length of time may be correlated with resolution of symptoms. To refine our analysis, we looked at the duration of care received for five diagnostic groups:

1. any diagnoses
2. behavioral health
3. symptoms commonly associated with mTBI
4. personal history of TBI (V15.52)
5. any TBI diagnosis (including PCS, personal history of TBI, and TBI of any severity).[1]

Within each group, we then examined the duration over which service members received treatment for the diagnoses of interest, identifying when a service member was no longer receiving treatment for the diagnosis of interest (i.e., when we did not observe any further treatment for the diagnosis through the end of the six-month observation period). We also identified service members who received no care related to the diagnosis of interest. This approach is an approximation of the duration of care received for the diagnosis of interest.

Table 6.1 presents our results, which show that the majority of service members receive health care for these conditions for no longer than 90 days following their mTBI diagnosis, and many do so for only a few days after the diagnosis. Notably, the majority of service members in the 2012 mTBI cohort did not receive any care for symptoms or conditions commonly

Table 6.1
Duration and Patterns of Care, by Type of Care

Care Pattern	% of 2012 mTBI Cohort				
	Any	Behavioral Health[a]	Common Symptoms[b]	TBI History (V15.52)	TBI (any severity), PCS, TBI History (V15.52)
Discontinued care before 90 days	**21.8**	**82.4**	**80.6**	**89.8**	**86.8**
No care	—	73.3	50.0	74.6	—
Discontinued after 1 day	7.9	2.0	13.9	5.0	61.9
Discontinued within 2–7 days	1.6	0.7	4.1	1.6	10.9
Discontinued within 8–14 days	1.0	0.5	1.4	1.0	2.8
Discontinued within 15–30 days	1.9	1.1	2.7	2.0	3.7
Discontinued within 31–90 days	9.5	4.7	8.4	5.6	7.5
Persistent care > 90 days	**78.2**	**17.6**	**19.4**	**10.2**	**13.2**
Continuous	25.3	3.1	1.7	1.0	2.2
Delayed 15–30 days	—	2.4	2.0	1.6	—
Delayed 31–90 days	—	3.8	3.2	2.2	—

NOTES: N = 16,378. The table shows that 5 percent of the cohort received a V15.52 diagnostic code (history of TBI) on the first day of treatment (day of diagnosis). We do not know why this is the case. Some possible explanations include coding error or a patient who had multiple visits on the day of diagnosis.
[a] Treatment with diagnostic codes for adjustment disorders, anxiety, depression, PTSD, or acute stress disorders.
[b] Treatment with diagnosis codes for hearing problems, dizziness/vertigo, headache, irritability, memory loss, sleep problems, and vision problems.

---

[1]   We included this group in the analysis to be inclusive of cases in which a provider may not record diagnostic codes according to DoD ICD-9 coding guidance for TBI (e.g., if the provider recorded a TBI diagnosis beyond the initial visit).

associated with mTBI. These findings confirm what has been found in clinical studies (Carroll et al., 2014; Lundin et al., 2006; McCrea, Guskiewicz, et al., 2003). Nearly 80 percent of the mTBI cohort received some care (for any condition) beyond 90 days of mTBI diagnosis.

Among those who received mTBI-related care for longer than 90 days, we identified those who received care continuously throughout the six months of observation. We also identified those who did not have any care for the diagnosis in the first two weeks or month but then began receiving care for that diagnosis and continued doing so through the end of the observation period. Overall, our findings regarding care received after 90 days agree with previous research: Ten to 20 percent of the mTBI cohort, the so-called "miserable minority," have treatment needs beyond three months (Hartlage, Durant-Wilson and Patch, 2001; Ruff, 2005). As we show in the remainder of this chapter and in Chapter Eight, service members with mTBI who continue to receive treatment for symptoms past three months use a significant amount of care.

Patterns of Care in the 2012 mTBI Cohort

To understand patterns of care among the 2012 mTBI cohort, we grouped care into 26 weekly increments after the mTBI diagnosis. This approach allowed us to observe a single week to examine whether any of the service members in the cohort received care at that time. It also allowed us to compare care use by week to see whether patterns changed over time. Figures 6.1–6.3 show trends over the six months following a new mTBI diagnosis.

Figure 6.1
Total Health Care Utilization Following mTBI Diagnosis, Weeks 1–26

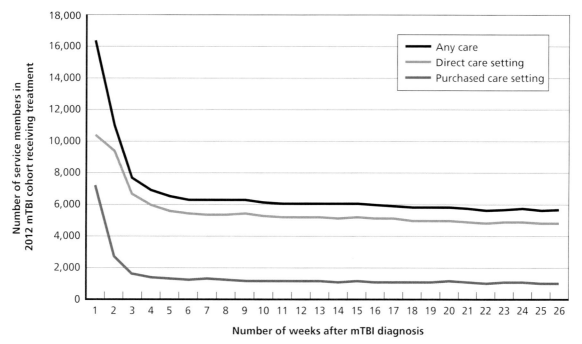

Figure 6.2
Health Care Utilization for Symptoms and Conditions Commonly Associated with mTBI, Weeks 1–26

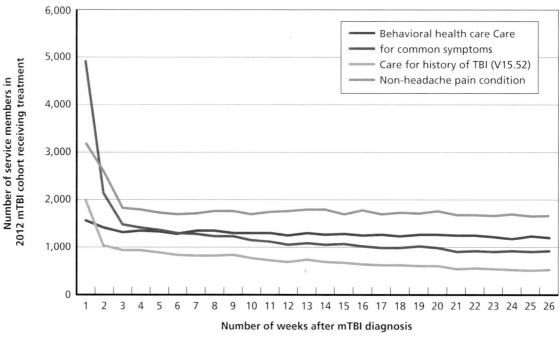

RAND RR844-6.2

Figure 6.3
Health Care Utilization for Symptoms and Conditions Commonly Associated with mTBI, Days 1–30

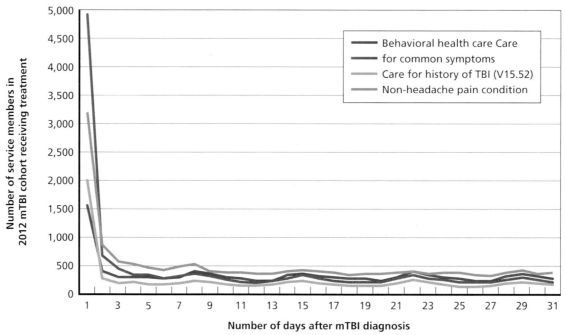

RAND RR844-6.3

Total Health Care Utilization, Weeks 1–26

In Figure 6.1, we plotted weekly utilization for three groups in the mTBI cohort: all service members, those receiving treatment through the direct care system, and those receiving treatment through the purchased care system. The first data point in Figure 6.1 is for care received on the same day as the mTBI diagnosis, and observations thereafter are for subsequent care received and shown in weekly (seven-day) increments.

Total utilization, represented by the black line, revealed a clear episode beginning but no clear episode end. All 16,378 service members in the 2012 mTBI cohort were included at the beginning, receiving care during the diagnostic visit for the mTBI. We observed a sharp drop from the first day of treatment through the following week, followed by a moderate drop from two to five weeks after the mTBI diagnosis. Utilization then dropped gradually from six weeks after the mTBI diagnosis through the end of the observation period of 25 weeks.

Health Care Utilization for Symptoms and Conditions Commonly Associated with mTBI, Weeks 1–26

In Figure 6.2, we plotted weekly utilization for all service members receiving care for symptoms and conditions that commonly co-occur with mTBI. We assessed four diagnostic groups: behavioral health care, care for common symptoms, care for personal history of TBI (V15.52), and care for non-headache pain conditions.[2] Here, again, the first observation is for the day of diagnosis only, and the 25 observations thereafter are shown in seven-day segments.

The figure shows strong patterns. About one-third of service members (n = 4,915) received treatment for common symptoms on the day of their mTBI diagnosis. This number dropped precipitously through week 2, when 1,488 service members (9 percent of the 2012 mTBI cohort) received care for common symptoms, and then continued to drop gradually through week 19, to 923 service members (6 percent), after which it remained flat. Care for service members with a personal history of TBI (V15.52) followed this same pattern, starting with 2,002 patients receiving care on day 1 (12 percent of the 2012 mTBI cohort), trailing off to 946 patients (6 percent) by week 2, and then declining gradually to 549 patients by week 19 and remaining flat after that.

Similarly, care for non-headache pain conditions dropped off quickly from weeks 1 to 3. One in five service members (n = 3,203, 20 percent of the 2012 mTBI cohort) received treatment for non-headache pain on the first day following an mTBI diagnosis. The number of service members receiving treatment for non-headache pain dropped in week 2 to 1,835 (11 percent), and from week 3 onward dropped off very slowly, appearing to level off by week 19 at around 1,700 service members (10 percent of the 2012 mTBI cohort). This pattern of rapid drop-off to nearly uniform utilization from weeks 3 through 25 suggests that non-headache pain may be a result of comorbid injuries sustained with the mTBI. The receipt of treatment for non-headache pain did not appear to resolve the symptoms as quickly as treatment for other conditions, and the number of service members receiving such care was consistently higher than any other diagnosis group we examined. The rate of treatment for non-headache pain in the weekly increments is not a prevalence of the condition per se, but it amounts to approximately 10 percent of service members receiving treatment each week.

The number of service members who received care for behavioral health conditions appeared to be relatively consistent over time. After a slight decline from day 1 to week 2 of

---

[2]   Headache pain is included among the common symptoms of mTBI.

1,568 (10 percent of the 2012 mTBI cohort) to 1,333 service members (8 percent of the cohort), the number of service members receiving behavioral health care was roughly uniform over the remaining 23 weeks, with between 7 and 8 percent of the mTBI cohort receiving care for behavioral health conditions in any given week. We interpret the uniform utilization line over this length of time as indicative of a baseline or underlying care pattern for behavioral health care in the mTBI cohort, suggesting that these may be primarily preexisting conditions.

Health Care Utilization for Symptoms and Conditions Commonly Associated with mTBI, Days 1–30

We observed patterns of care over 25 weeks, but we also examined care for the same diagnostic groups over each day in the first 30 days following the mTBI diagnosis to identify any details that may have been obscured by the weekly analysis (see Figure 6.3). We found that during the first week after mTBI diagnosis, 10–20 percent of service members received care associated with common symptoms of mTBI, personal history of TBI, behavioral health, and non-headache pain, and a large majority of care observed during the first week was provided on the same day as the mTBI diagnosis.

Conclusions

This chapter presented findings on the duration and patterns of care among active-duty, non-deployed service members in the six months after an mTBI diagnosis, illustrating several key trends. First, most service members in the 2012 mTBI cohort received health care for diagnoses potentially related to the mTBI for less than four weeks. Most service members received any TBI-relevant care within the first week after diagnosis, with slower but still substantial further reductions from two to five weeks and only modest reductions after six weeks. Second, care continued for a small group of service members through three months. The total proportion of service members who received care past one month was 15–30 percent of the cohort. Between 3 and 10 percent of service members received care through three months but did not receive care beyond that time. Finally, care continued for an even smaller group through six months.

CHAPTER SEVEN

What Types of Care Do Nondeployed Active-Duty Service Members with mTBI Receive in the Six Months After Their mTBI Diagnosis?

In this chapter, we describe the diagnostic assessments, therapies, and medications received by the 2012 mTBI cohort in the six months following their mTBI diagnosis. The most recommended initial treatment for mTBI is rest and patient education, activities that were not observable in the health care utilization data. However, some patients with mTBI receive care beyond the initial visit; as such, we report on diagnostic assessments and treatments received by the mTBI cohort in the six months following the mTBI diagnosis. We caution that we were not able to determine whether the care received by service members in the 2012 mTBI cohort was for the mTBI or for another condition. Current TBI coding guidance recommends that health care visits after the initial visit include symptom diagnostic codes rather than a TBI-related diagnostic code. As such, it is not possible to know whether physical therapy, for example, was related to the mTBI or a different condition. Our analysis was conducted with this constraint, but we offer suggestions for possible changes and improvements in coding guidance in Chapter Nine.

VA/DoD clinical practice guidelines suggest that, immediately following a concussion or brain injury, providers should complete a thorough evaluation of the patient's medical history and a physical examination. Providers should also initiate conservative management with a 24-hour rest period, during which the patient is instructed to limit physical and mental activity and remain in a low-stimulus environment (VA and DoD, 2009). Over the following days, providers should monitor symptoms and recovery with increases in activity based on the patient's recovery; typically, this process lasts one week. During this acute phase of the injury, the guidelines also recommend providing reassurance and positive expectations of full recovery, as well as patient education about mTBI, including sleep hygiene, relaxation, and other supportive care recommendations, such as proper nutrition and fluid intake.

If symptoms persist, the guidelines recommend that providers continue thorough evaluation but may consider further testing, such as neuroimaging (CT or MRI). Subsequent treatment is typically symptom-focused. For example, treatment and management of headaches may include patient education on neck stretches, treating underlying conditions (such as poor sleep), aerobic exercise, relaxation training, physical therapy, and pharmacological intervention for extreme headaches. For dizziness and disequilibrium, treatment may include vestibular and balance rehabilitation. For fatigue and sleep symptoms, treatment may include patient education, sleep hygiene, or medication. For behavioral health problems, treatment is condition-specific but may include psychotherapy or medication.

Diagnostic Assessments

In Table 7.1, we describe the proportion of the mTBI cohort who received various diagnostic assessments and evaluations within the six months following their mTBI diagnosis. As the table shows, one-third of the cohort received a CT scan, 29 percent received a psychiatric diagnostic evaluation, and 25 percent received a physical therapy evaluation. Smaller proportions of the cohort received a neuropsychological assessment (11 percent), a sleep study (5 percent), and other assessments.

Figure 7.1 shows the frequency of diagnostic assessments and evaluations in the six months following mTBI diagnosis by TBI history. For almost every assessment or evaluation, service members who had a previous TBI (of any severity) were more likely to receive the assessment or evaluation in the six months following their mTBI diagnosis, compared with service members who did not have a previous TBI (p < 0.001).

Therapies and Treatments for Symptoms and Conditions That Commonly or Occasionally Co-Occur with mTBI

Table 7.2 shows the proportion of the mTBI cohort who received various therapies and other treatments, for whatever reason, in the six months following the mTBI diagnosis. As is illustrated in the table, 30 percent received psychotherapy, mostly individual psychotherapy.

Table 7.1
Diagnostic Assessments and Evaluations Received in the Six Months After mTBI Diagnosis

Diagnostic Assessments	Number	% of 2012 mTBI Cohort
CT scan	5,398	33.0
Psychiatric diagnostic evaluation	4,705	28.7
Physical therapy evaluation	4,058	24.8
Neuropsychological assessment	1,829	11.2
Audiology examination	1,689	10.3
Occupational therapy evaluation	1,578	9.6
Health and behavior assessment	1,459	8.9
Neurobehavioral status exam	1,253	7.7
Evaluation of speech, language, voice, communication, or auditory processing	896	5.5
Sleep study	772	4.7
Sensorimotor examination	442	2.7
Vestibular testing	356	2.2

NOTES: N = 16,378. Assessments and evaluations may be related to co-occurring conditions rather than mTBI.

Figure 7.1
Diagnostic Assessments and Evaluations Received in the Six Months After mTBI Diagnosis, by TBI History

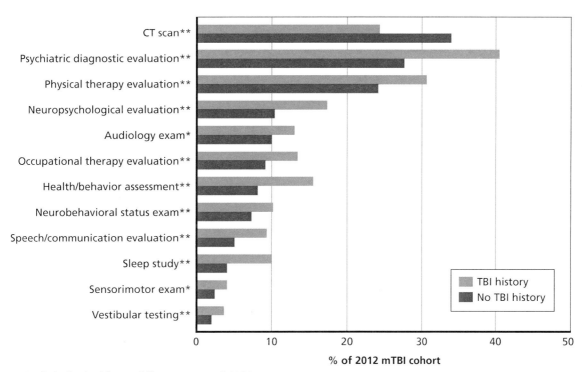

** Statistically significant difference at p < 0.0001.
 * Statistically significant difference at p < 0.001.
RAND *RR844-7.1*

Almost 25 percent received physical therapy, 10 percent received some form of complementary and alternative medicine (CAM), and smaller proportions received other treatments.

Because service members could have been receiving these therapies before the mTBI diagnosis, we examined the proportion of the mTBI cohort who received treatment both before and after the mTBI diagnosis, indicating ongoing care for a condition unrelated to the mTBI, compared with those who received treatment only after the mTBI diagnosis (see Figure 7.2). For most of the therapies and treatments we examined, relatively few (10 to 25 percent) of those who received treatment in the six months after the mTBI diagnosis had received the same treatment in the six months prior to the mTBI diagnosis. About half of those who received psychotherapy after the mTBI diagnosis also received psychotherapy before the mTBI diagnosis.

Similar to our findings related to diagnostic assessments and evaluations, we found that service members who had a previous TBI were more likely to receive various forms of treatment (see Figure 7.3; all differences were statistically significant, p < 0.0001). In particular, service members with a previous TBI were much more likely to receive psychotherapy in the six months following their 2012 mTBI diagnosis (44 percent) compared with service members who did not have a previous TBI (28 percent).

Table 7.2
Therapies Received, for Any Reason, in the Six Months Following Initial mTBI Diagnosis

Therapy/Treatment Type	Number	% of 2012 mTBI Cohort
Psychotherapy (any)	4,851	29.6
Individual psychotherapy	4,577	27.9
Group psychotherapy	1,372	8.4
Family psychotherapy	384	2.3
Physical therapy (therapeutic exercise, neuromuscular reeducation, physical therapy activities)	3,882	23.7
CAM (any)	1,675	10.2
Acupuncture	287	1.8
Chiropractic	722	4.4
Biofeedback	232	1.4
Other CAM	751	4.6
Occupational therapy	1,242	7.6
Neuromuscular electrical stimulation	1,175	7.2
Speech therapy	1,059	6.5
Cognitive rehabilitation	862	5.3
Health and behavior intervention	608	3.7
Positive airway pressure devices[a]	336	2.1
Sensory integration therapy	149	0.9

NOTES: N = 16,378. Treatments may be related to co-occurring conditions rather than mTBI.

[a] These devices include both continuous positive airway pressure (CPAP) and bilevel positive airway pressure (BiPAP) machines.

Medications

Medication treatment was common among the 2012 mTBI cohort, with 88 percent filling at least one prescription, for any reason, in the six months after the mTBI diagnosis. Many service members filled multiple prescriptions over this period, filling an average of 9.5 prescriptions in the six months following diagnosis. We note that a given medication can be prescribed for multiple conditions, depending on provider judgment, so it is not possible to know why (for what conditions) these medications were prescribed.

Figure 7.4 shows the proportion of the 2012 mTBI cohort who filled at least one prescription for medications commonly used for symptoms or conditions associated with mTBI in the six months following the mTBI diagnosis. The figure also indicates the proportion of those who also filled a prescription for that medication in the six months before the mTBI diagnosis.

Figure 7.2
Therapies and Treatment, for Any Cause, in the Six Months Before and After mTBI Diagnosis

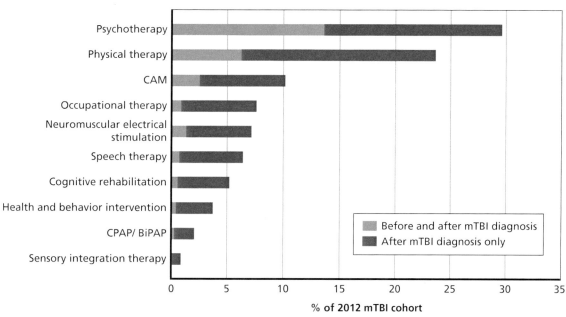

RAND RR844-7.2

Figure 7.3
Therapies Received in the Six Months After mTBI Diagnosis, by TBI History

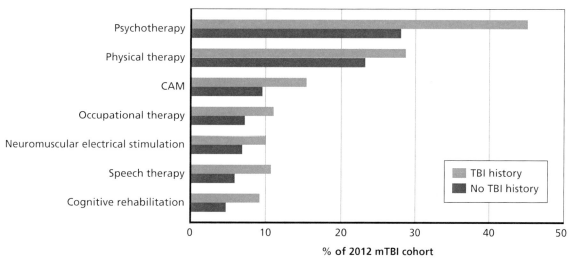

NOTES: Treatments may be related to co-occurring conditions rather than mTBI. All differences statistically significant at p < 0.0001.
RAND RR844-7.3

As is illustrated in the figure, 62 percent of the mTBI cohort filled a prescription for an analgesic in the six months following their mTBI diagnosis. Of these service members, half also filled a prescription for an analgesic in the six months before their mTBI diagnosis.

Almost half (45 percent) filled a prescription for an opioid in the six months after the mTBI diagnosis, and a quarter (24 percent) filled a prescription for an antidepressant. A third

Figure 7.4
Prescriptions Filled in the Six Months Before and After mTBI Diagnosis

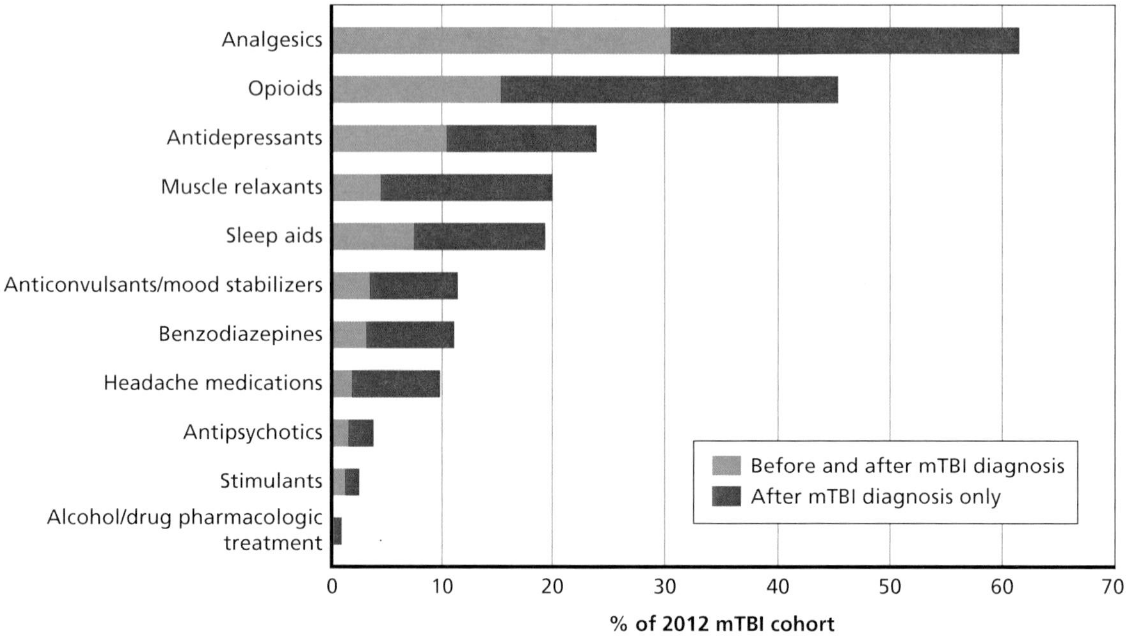

NOTE: Analgesics include NSAIDs, acetaminophen, and other non-opioid analgesics.
RAND *RR844-7.4*

of those who filled a prescription for an opioid and almost half of those who filled a prescription for an antidepressant also filled a prescription for these medications in the six months before the mTBI diagnosis.

To better understand the use of medications by this cohort, we examined the prescriptions filled by service members with an mTBI diagnosis who received treatment for headache, sleep disorders, or PTSD (see Figure 7.5). Many nondeployed active-duty service members with mTBI and co-occurring PTSD filled prescriptions in the six months following the mTBI diagnosis (e.g., 56 percent with mTBI and PTSD filled a prescription for an opioid). We found that 33 percent of those with mTBI and PTSD filled a prescription for benzodiazepines; VA/DoD treatment guidelines for PTSD recommend against the use of benzodiazepine in this population (VA and DoD, 2010). Three-quarters of service members with mTBI and PTSD filled a prescription for an antidepressant, compared with 55 percent of those receiving treatment for sleep disorders and 40 percent of those receiving treatment for headache.

We observed few differences between service members with a history of TBI and those without a previous TBI in the use of certain medications, such as analgesics and opioids (see Figure 7.6). However, those with a history of TBI were more likely than those without a previous TBI to have filled a prescription for an antidepressant, sleep aid, mood stabilizer, or other medications (p < 0.001). Specifically, 38 percent of those with a history of TBI filled a prescription for an antidepressant, compared with 22 percent of those without a previous TBI (p < 0.0001). This likely reflects the differences between these groups in terms of the prevalence of depression, as discussed in Chapter Four.

Figure 7.5
Prescriptions Filled in the Six Months After mTBI Diagnosis, by Co-Occurring Diagnoses

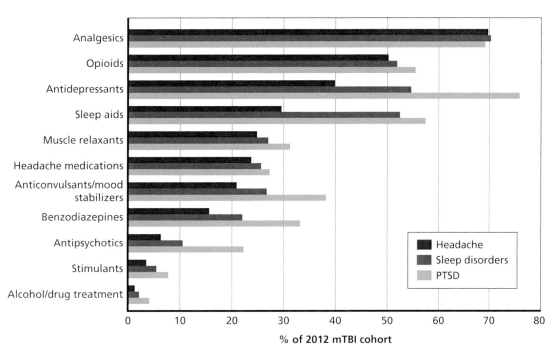

NOTES: Service members are counted in each applicable condition category. For instance, someone who has both headaches and PTSD will be included in both categories. Analgesics include NSAIDs, acetaminophen, and other non-opioid analgesics.
RAND RR844-7.5

Conclusions

This chapter reported the diagnostic assessments, therapies, and medications received by the 2012 mTBI cohort in the six months after diagnosis. In interpreting these results, it is important to note that, after the initial mTBI diagnosis, the data do not allow us to determine whether a visit (and the associated assessments, therapies, and medications) is specifically for mTBI or for another condition; much of the treatment described in this chapter could have been for conditions unrelated to the mTBI.

The most common diagnostic assessment received by those in the mTBI cohort was a CT scan; one-third received a CT scan in the six months following diagnosis. Psychiatric diagnostic evaluations and physical therapy evaluations were also common, with 30 percent and 25 percent of the mTBI cohort receiving them, respectively. Service members who had a history of TBI at the time of the mTBI diagnosis were more likely than those without a TBI history to receive most of the diagnostic assessments.

Of the therapies and specific treatments received by the mTBI cohort in the six months after the mTBI diagnosis, the most common were psychotherapy (especially individual psychotherapy) and physical therapy. As with diagnostic assessments, those who had a history of TBI or deployment at the time of diagnosis were more likely than those without to receive most of the therapies we considered.

Figure 7.6
Prescriptions Filled in the Six Months After mTBI Diagnosis, by TBI History

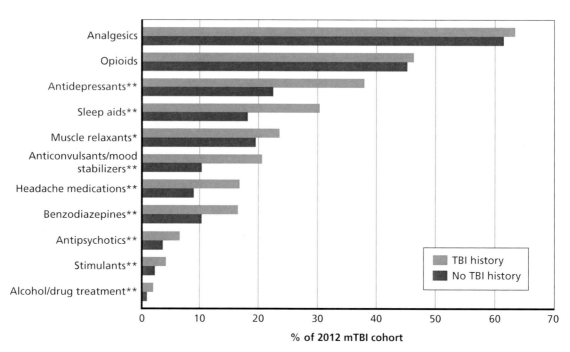

NOTES: Prescriptions may be related to co-occurring conditions rather than mTBI. Analgesics include NSAIDs, acetaminophen, and other non-opioid analgesics.
**Statistically significant difference at p < 0.0001.
*Statistically significant difference at p < 0.001.
RAND RR844-7.6

Finally, we explored the types of prescriptions filled by mTBI cohort in the six months following diagnosis, the most common of which were analgesics, opioids, and antidepressants, filled by half, one-third, and one-quarter of the cohort, respectively. Service members in the mTBI cohort who had a history of TBI at the time of mTBI diagnosis were more likely than their counterparts with no history of TBI to fill some prescriptions, most notably antidepressants, sleep aids, and mood stabilizers. Finally, we considered whether the rate of filled prescriptions varied by three commonly co-occurring conditions: headaches, sleep disorders, and PTSD. All prescriptions (except analgesics, which were filled nearly equally by mTBI cohort members with each of the three co-occurring conditions) were most commonly filled by those whose mTBI was co-occurring with PTSD.

CHAPTER EIGHT

Who Receives Persistent Care Following mTBI Diagnosis?

As we discussed in Chapter Six, most service members in the 2012 mTBI cohort received no or only short-term treatment for symptoms and co-occurring conditions after their mTBI diagnosis, suggesting that they recovered quickly. However, a sizable minority (10–20 percent) continued to receive care for three months or more after the mTBI diagnosis.

According to ICD-9 and DSM-IV diagnostic criteria, many of these individuals should be classified as having PCS. Clinically, PCS is defined by a cluster of physical symptoms that persist for three months or more after a concussion. The symptoms include headache, dizziness, fatigue, visual disturbances, noise and light sensitivity, memory deficits, attention, concentration and executive function deficits, depression, and anxiety (Ryan and Warden, 2003). It should be acknowledged that while it is widely agreed that patients with PCS suffer from the aforementioned physical symptoms, there is debate about the exact combination of symptoms that constitute the disorder (Dean, O'Neill, and Sterr, 2012) and whether the cluster of symptoms should even constitute a separate disorder (Lagarde et al., 2014).

Although we might have expected to observe PCS diagnoses in our data on service members in the 2012 mTBI cohort who received mTBI-related treatment for more than three months after the mTBI diagnosis, we found that only 6.6 percent had a PCS diagnosis in the six-month observation window, compared with the 10–20 percent of the cohort receiving care for more than three months. Since this finding suggests that the PCS diagnostic code may undercount the subpopulation experiencing ongoing problems related to mTBI, we used two approaches to identify and describe the population of service members with persistent care needs.

- First, we identified service members in the 2012 mTBI cohort who received treatment reported with a secondary diagnostic code for personal history of TBI (V15.52) treatment that lasted longer than 90 days (three months) after the initial mTBI diagnosis (hereafter, persistent care).
- Second, we identified all service members who received a PCS diagnosis in 2012, regardless of whether they had an mTBI diagnosis. We constructed this separate cohort to identify a broader group of service members with potential ongoing care needs related to mTBI. These service members may have had a head injury that occurred prior to the study period, or they never received an mTBI diagnosis because they did not seek care for the acute injury. It is worth noting that just 32 percent of service members with a PCS diagnosis in 2012 had a TBI diagnosis of any severity in the six months prior to the PCS diagnosis.

This chapter first compares the differences in demographic characteristics, utilization of care, and comorbid conditions between those who required persistent care and those who did not in the 2012 mTBI cohort. Then, it explores the demographic and service characteristics of the population of service members receiving treatment for PCS in 2012.

Characteristics of Nondeployed Active-Duty Service Members Who Received Persistent Care

We identified 1,678 service members who received persistent care. Table 8.1 compares the demographic and service characteristics of service members who did and did not receive persistent care, as well as the relative risks for receiving persistent care. We adjusted this relative risk to account for potential confounding variables, such as sex, service branch, and deployment history.

We found that having had a previous TBI is predictive of persistent care after a new mTBI diagnosis. A service member in the 2012 mTBI cohort was almost 50 percent more likely to receive persistent care if he or she had a previous TBI (p < 0.0001). This finding is consistent with the findings of Guskiewicz et al. (2005), who demonstrated that a previous mTBI is a risk factor for having trouble recovering from subsequent mTBIs. It is unclear from our data, however, whether increased persistent health care use was due solely to the previous mTBI or other mitigating variables, such as behavioral health problems or increased selection by medical personnel for continued monitoring. Despite this, there is a clearly a strong statistical relationship.

We did not find a significant relationship between sex and persistent care. This differs from the findings of Guinto and Guinto-Nishimura (2014), Bazarian and Atabaki (2001), and Farace and Alves (2000), all of whom found that women are at a higher risk of developing persistent problems after an mTBI. This could be explained by the robust relationship between a previous TBI diagnosis and persistent care. In the military context, men are more likely to be exposed to combat and TBI than women, potentially reducing the impact of sex on the development of persistent problems.

We also detected an increased risk for individuals older than 35; this group was 33 percent more likely to receive persistent care than those ages 18–34 (p < 0.01). This finding is consistent with the findings of Packard, Weaver, and Ham (1993) and Fenton et al. (1993), who demonstrated that age is a risk factor for developing ongoing TBI-related problems. It is unclear from these data, however, whether this is due to changes in the brain as it ages or some other mitigating variable, such as differences in health-seeking behavior as individuals age.

We also found significant differences in the rates of persistent care by marital status. Having never been married was associated with a lower rate of persistent care, whereas divorcees and widowers were 24 percent more likely to seek care for persistent problems than the other marital statuses combined. An important element of recovering from an mTBI is proper support both at work and at home, and this support may be less available to those who are divorced or widowed.

We also observed differences in rates of persistent care by TRICARE region, with a significantly higher rate in the TRICARE West region. While potentially important, the reasons for this difference are unclear. One hypothesis is that coding guidance may not be consistent across regions.

Table 8.1
Adjusted Relative Risk for Receiving Persistent Care Among Service Members with a Personal History of TBI, by Demographic and Service Characteristics

Characteristic	Persistent Care Number	%	No Persistent Care Number	%	Total Number	%	Adjusted Relative Risk	Confidence Interval
Sex								
Male	1,548	92.3	12,654	86.1	14,202	86.7	1.18	0.98–1.42
Female	130	7.7	2,046	13.9	2,176	13.3	0.85	0.70–1.03
Age at diagnosis								
18–34	1,352	80.6	12,666	86.1	14018	85.6	0.75	0.59–0.96*
35 or older	326	19.4	2,033	13.8	2359	14.4	1.33	1.05–1.69*
Race/ethnicity								
White, non-Hispanic	1,165	69.4	9,534	64.9	10,699	65.3	1.03	0.89–1.18
Black, non-Hispanic	190	11.3	2,129	14.5	2,319	14.2	0.79	0.66–0.96***
Hispanic	200	11.9	1,643	11.2	1,843	11.3	0.97	0.80–1.16
Other/unknown	123	7.3	1,394	9.5	1,517	9.3	1.14	0.92–1.41
Marital Status								
Married	1,160	69.1	7,989	54.3	9,149	55.9	1.12	0.98–1.27
Never married	422	25.1	6,022	41.0	6,444	39.3	0.72	0.62–0.84***
Divorced, separated, or widowed	96	5.7	682	4.6	778	4.8	1.24	1.00–1.54*
Region								
TRICARE North	431	25.8	3,990	27.1	4,421	27.0	1.14	0.95–1.37
TRICARE South	258	15.4	3,077	20.9	3,335	20.4	0.90	0.74–1.10
TRICARE West	821	49.1	6,109	41.5	6,930	42.3	1.26	1.06–1.49**
TRICARE Overseas	150	9.0	1,388	9.4	1,539	9.4	1.17	0.94–1.45
TBI history (V15.52)	294	17.5	1,317	9.0	1,611	9.8	1.48	1.30–1.68***
Service branch								
Army	1,306	77.8	7,485	50.9	8,791	53.7	3.75	2.74–5.14***
Navy	60	3.6	2,131	14.5	2,191	13.4	0.71	0.48–1.05
Air Force	46	2.7	2,640	18.0	2,686	16.4	0.41	0.27–0.61***
Marine Corps	261	15.6	1,987	13.5	2,248	13.7	3.74	2.70–5.18***
Other/unknown	5	0.3	457	3.1	462	2.8	0.25	0.08–0.77**
Deployment history	1,496	89.2	9,361	63.7	10,857	66.3	2.50	2.08–2.99***

NOTES: TBI history is defined by ICD-9 code V15.52. Persistent care is defined as treatment associated with a personal history of mTBI for 90 days or more after mTBI diagnosis. Relative risk is adjusted for gender, age, race, marital status, TRICARE region, TBI history, service branch, cumulative months of deployment, years of service, and deployment history. Numbers may not sum due to missing data.
*** Statistically significant difference at $p < 0.001$
** Statistically significant difference at $p < 0.01$
* Statistically significant difference at $p < 0.05$

Service members in our cohort who had been deployed were two and a half times more likely to receive persistent care compared with those who did not have a history of deployment (p < 0.0001). It is also notable that Army and Marine Corps personnel were almost four times as likely to receive persistent care than Navy and Air Force personnel (p < 0.0001). One hypothesis is that soldiers and marines have occupational specialties that exposed them to more risk factors for long-term treatment needs, such as multiple TBIs (Guskiewicz et al., 2005) and PTSD, which are commonly comorbid and cause ongoing problems. Alternatively, this difference might be attributable to differences in coding practices across service branches.

We found higher rates of comorbid mental health conditions among service members in the 2012 mTBI cohort who received persistent care than among those who did not receive persistent care (see Figure 8.1). Just under 40 percent of those who received persistent care had also received treatment for PTSD, compared with 8 percent of those who did not receive persistent care. This is consistent with the findings of Brenner et al. (2010) and Schneiderman, Braver, and Kang (2008), who found that PTSD increased the likelihood of persistent postconcussive symptoms among military personnel. Similarly, 29 percent of those who received persistent care received treatment for depression, compared with 11 percent of those who did not receive persistent care. We also found that the proportion who received treatment for alcohol abuse and dependence was slightly higher among those who did not receive persistent care than among those who did. We remind the reader that these data merely demonstrate the co-occurrence of these disorders and do not, in themselves, establish a causal relationship between mental illness and ongoing symptoms or conditions commonly associated with mTBI. There is the potential that those with mental health conditions have increased contact with medical professionals and, as a result, are diagnosed with ongoing problems at a higher rate. Fur-

Figure 8.1
Co-Occurring Behavioral Health Conditions Among Service Members with mTBI Diagnosis, by Duration of Treatment

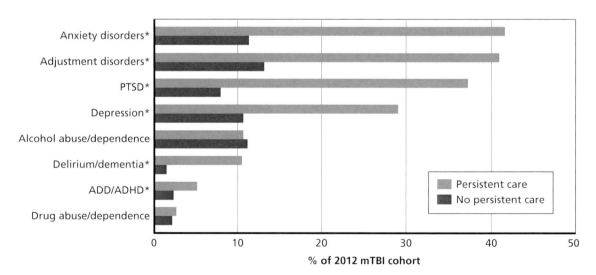

NOTES: Persistent care is defined as treatment associated with a personal history of mTBI for 90 days or more after mTBI diagnosis. TBI history is defined by ICD-9 code V15.52. Anxiety disorders include generalized anxiety disorder, OCD, anxiety not otherwise specified, and panic disorder. Depression includes major depressive disorder and dysthymia.

*Statistically significant difference at p < 0.0001.

RAND RR844-8.1

thermore, these analyses only demonstrate co-occurrence, not which diagnosis (if either) was received first.

Figure 8.2 illustrates the prevalence of co-occurring symptoms and conditions among those who did and did not receive persistent care. It is important to note that these individuals may have received treatment for these symptoms and conditions at any time during the six-month observation period. We found a high rate of these symptoms and conditions among those who received persistent care compared with those who did not. Of note, almost three-quarters of those with persistent care needs received treatment for memory loss compared with less than 10 percent of those who did not receive persistent care (p < 0.0001). Treatment for sleep disorders, headaches, and dizziness was also more common among those with persistent care needs than among those without long-term problems (p < 0.0001). While these were the conditions with the largest differences in rates between the two groups, service members with persistent care needs received treatment more often for each condition in Figure 8.2 than did those without persistent care needs, except for syncope/collapse.

Figures 8.3–8.5 show that those with persistent care needs received more diagnostic assessments and therapies and filled more prescriptions in the six months following their mTBI diagnosis than those who did not receive persistent care. (All differences were statistically significant, p < 0.0001.) It is to be expected that those with long-term problems stemming from

Figure 8.2
Co-Occurring Symptoms and Conditions Among Service Members with mTBI Diagnosis, by Duration of Treatment

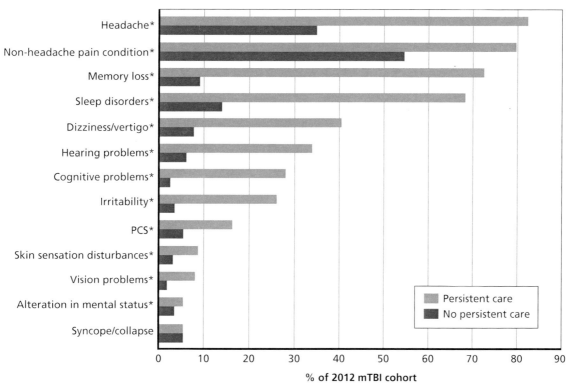

NOTES: Persistent care is defined as treatment associated with a personal history of mTBI for 90 days or more after mTBI diagnosis. TBI history is defined by ICD-9 code V15.52.

*Statistically significant difference at p < 0.0001.

RAND RR844-8.2

mTBI would be more engaged with the health care system, but some findings related to health care utilization may be particularly significant.

Figure 8.3 illustrates differences in the receipt of diagnostic assessments and evaluations between those with persistent care needs and those without. Service members with persistent care needs received psychiatric evaluations, physical therapy evaluations, and occupational therapy evaluations at a rate more than three times that of those without long-term problems. The rate was more than twice as high in almost every other category. Interestingly, CT scan rates were higher among those without persistent care needs.

Figure 8.4 shows differences in the use of behavioral health services between those who did and did not receive persistent care. While just one-quarter of service members in the mTBI cohort without persistent care needs received psychotherapy in the six months following the mTBI diagnosis, nearly 80 percent of those with long-term problems received psychotherapy. Psychotherapy is one recommended course of therapy for those who develop PCS, so it may not be surprising that those with long-term issues related to mTBI would receive this type of treatment (Reddy, 2011). In addition, service members with persistent care needs frequently had co-occurring mental health conditions, which may also explain this finding. We found that those with persistent care needs received speech therapy and cognitive rehabilitation at a rate about eight times the rate of those without long-term problems. Finally, a minority of those with persistent care needs (just under 10 percent) received sensory integration therapy, but almost none of the service members without ongoing care needs did so.

Figure 8.3
Diagnostic Assessments Among Service Members with mTBI Diagnosis

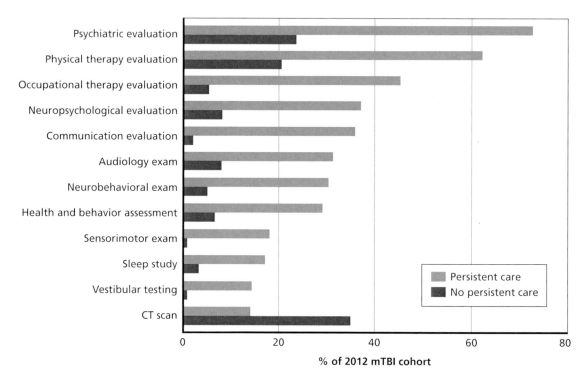

NOTES: Persistent care is defined as treatment associated with a personal history of mTBI for 90 days or more after mTBI diagnosis. TBI history is defined by ICD-9 code V15.52. All differences statistically significant at p < 0.0001.
RAND RR844-8.3

Figure 8.4
Therapies in the Six Months After mTBI Diagnosis Among Service Members with mTBI Diagnosis

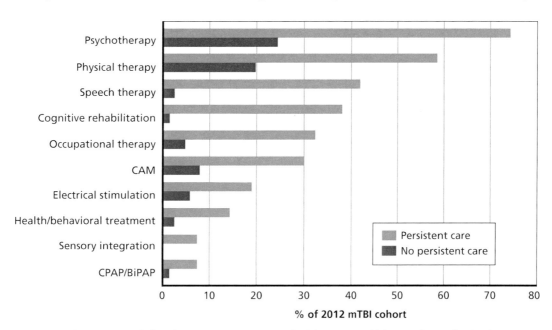

NOTES: Persistent care is defined as treatment associated with a personal history of mTBI for 90 days or more after mTBI diagnosis. TBI history is defined by ICD-9 code V15.52. Therapies may be related to co-occurring conditions rather than mTBI. All differences statistically significant at p < 0.0001.
RAND RR844-8.4

Figure 8.5 illustrates differences by persistent care in terms of medication use. While 67 percent of those with persistent care needs filled a prescription for an antidepressant, just 19 percent of those without did so. Similarly, 50 percent of those with persistent care needs filled a prescription for a sleep aid, compared with 16 percent of those without long-term treatment. This pattern was repeated for each medication type, with a much larger proportion of those with persistent care needs filling prescriptions.

In this section, we describe the characteristics of service members who received treatment associated with PCS in 2012. Recall from Chapter Two that this population is likely related to, but different from, the persistent care population described in this chapter. Service members with PCS received a diagnosis indicative of long-term, persistent problems subsequent to mTBI, while the population described here received long-term care but, in most cases, did not receive a PCS diagnosis. One goal of this section is to explicitly compare the differences between the PCS cohort and the empirically derived cohort with persistent care needs described earlier in this chapter.

Table 8.2 shows the demographic characteristics of the service members who received a PCS diagnosis in 2012. The data indicate that these service members were overwhelmingly male and mostly white, non-Hispanic, largely reflecting the demographic composition of the military as a whole. Interestingly, the majority of those with PCS were between the ages of 25 and 34—older than might have been expected, given that the largest age group of service members is under 25 years old. One possible explanation for this finding is that having had multiple TBIs is a risk factor for PCS (Guskiewicz et al., 2005), and it may be that older service members have more exposure over their careers to situations in which they are at risk of a

Figure 8.5
Prescriptions Filled in the Six Months After mTBI Diagnosis Among Service Members Diagnosed with mTBI

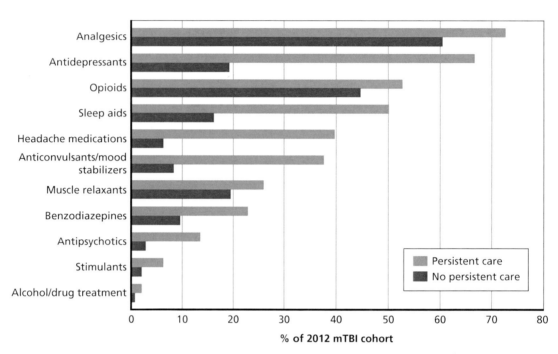

NOTES: Persistent care is defined as treatment associated with a personal history of mTBI for 90 days or more after mTBI diagnosis. TBI history is defined by ICD-9 code V15.52. Analgesics include NSAIDs, acetaminophen, and other non-opioid analgesics. All differences statistically significant at p < 0.0001.
RAND RR844-8.5

head injury. Alternatively, this finding may reflect the fact that age has been found to be a risk factor for post-concussive symptoms (Fenton et al., 1993; Packard, Weaver, and Ham, 1993).

A large majority of service members with PCS were married, which may be due to the fact that the group is also slightly older than the military as a whole. Finally, about a quarter of the group (26 percent) had a previous TBI between 2008 and 2011. As previously stated, multiple TBIs are a risk factor for PCS (Guskiewicz et al., 2005).

Table 8.3 shows the service characteristics of the cohort of service members who received treatment associated with PCS in 2012. As in the overall military, the majority of those with PCS were Army personnel. Notably, however, only 10 percent of those with PCS were marines. While the Marine Corps is a smaller force, its personnel are at a high risk of head injury, so this result is somewhat surprising. There may be differences in diagnosing and coding PCS by service, however.

Most of those with PCS (80 percent) had a history of deployment. This likely increased their exposure to combat trauma, including head injuries, and increased their risk for other comorbid conditions often associated with PCS, such as PTSD (Brenner et al., 2010; Lagarde et al., 2014; Schneiderman, Braver, and Kang, 2008) and anxiety (Fenton et al., 1993).

We also examined the extent to which service members who received treatment associated with PCS also received treatment for co-occurring conditions. Table 8.4 describes the proportion of those with PCS who received treatment for selected conditions and diagnoses in the six months following their first health care encounter for PCS in 2012. A large proportion

Table 8.2
Demographic Characteristics of Service Members
Receiving Treatment for PCS in 2012

Demographic Characteristics	Number	%
Sex		
Male	3,952	88.9
Female	491	11.1
Age at diagnosis		
18–24	1,574	35.4
25–34	1,917	43.1
35–44	825	18.6
45–64	127	2.9
Race/ethnicity		
White, non-Hispanic	3,072	69.1
Black, non-Hispanic	499	11.2
Hispanic	471	10.6
Asian or Pacific Islander	175	3.9
American Indian/Alaskan Native	76	1.7
Other/unknown	150	3.4
Marital status		
Married	2,938	66.1
Never married	1,255	28.2
Divorced, separated, widowed	250	5.6
Region		
TRICARE North	1,729	39.0
TRICARE South	986	22.2
TRICARE West	1,145	25.8
TRICARE Overseas	548	12.3
TBI history	1,175	26.4

NOTES: N = 4,443. TBI history is defined by ICD-9 code
V15.52. Numbers may not sum due to missing data.

Table 8.3
Service Characteristics of Service Members Receiving Treatment Associated with PCS in 2012

Service History Characteristics	Number	%
Service branch		
Army	2,624	59.1
Navy	942	21.2
Marine Corps	444	10.0
Air Force	349	7.9
Coast Guard	84	1.9
Rank at diagnosis		
E1–E4	2,000	45.0
E5–E9	2,022	45.5
O1–O3	208	4.7
O4–O6	107	2.4
Other/unknown	106	2.4
Years of service (mean)	7.8	—
Deployment history	3,576	80.5

NOTE: N = 4,443.

(55 percent) of those with PCS also received treatment for PTSD. It has been suggested in the literature that PCS and PTSD may not be separate conditions and that those with PCS may actually have PTSD (Lagarde et al., 2014). However, this assertion has not been well established by other research, which has instead demonstrated that comorbid conditions are common among those who experience PCS (Fenton et al., 1993; Ponsford et al., 2000; Thornhill et al., 2000). Our findings echo this research: More than 30 percent of our PCS cohort received treatment for an anxiety disorder, and nearly 30 percent received treatment for depression.

It may not be surprising that almost 65 percent of those with PCS received treatment for headache. Headache is one of the main symptoms of PCS, along with dizziness and memory loss, for which many service members with PCS also received treatment. We found that two-thirds of those with PCS received treatment for non-headache pain. This is a unique finding because non-headache pain has not previously been found to be comorbid with PCS. Pain could have a direct impact on the course of treatment for PCS patients, so this is an important finding for clinical care. At the very least, these comorbid conditions may complicate the diagnosis of PCS.

Table 8.4
Co-Occurring Conditions Among Service Members Receiving Treatment Associated with PCS in 2012

Co-Occurring Condition	Number	%
Behavioral health diagnoses		
PTSD	2,431	54.7
Anxiety disorders	1,396	31.4
Adjustment disorders	1,282	28.9
Depression	1,277	28.7
Delirium/dementia	533	12.0
Alcohol abuse/dependence	386	8.7
ADD/ADHD	233	5.2
Drug abuse/dependence	148	3.3
Acute stress disorders	71	1.6
Bipolar disorder	72	1.6
Associated diagnoses and symptoms		
Non-headache pain condition	3,027	68.1
Headache	2,848	64.1
Sleep disorders and symptoms	2,296	51.7
Memory loss	1,628	36.6
Dizziness/vertigo	1,084	24.4
Hearing problems	844	19.0
Cognitive problems	786	17.7
Skin sensation disturbances	304	6.8
Communication disorders (unrelated to development)	267	6.0
Syncope and collapse	213	4.8
Vision problems	184	4.1
Alteration in mental status	137	3.1
Gait and coordination problems	137	3.1
Irritability	311	7.0

NOTES: N = 4,443. Anxiety disorders include generalized anxiety disorder, OCD, anxiety not otherwise specified, and panic disorder. Depression includes major depressive disorder and dysthymia.

Conclusions

While we found that the majority of service members with mTBI recovered quickly from their injuries, there was a small group that continued to receive mTBI-related treatment for three months or more. Across many characteristics, those who needed persistent care were different from the majority of service members who were diagnosed with an mTBI, and they used significantly more health services than their counterparts without long-term problems. Those with persistent care needs may have long-term health problems and should be a target for future research.

Among those who received persistent care and those who received treatment associated with PCS, there was a high prevalence of co-occurring behavioral health problems, as well as headache, non-headache pain, and sleep problems. While these findings are descriptive, they provide useful information as a first step in understanding treatment needs for persistent symptoms subsequent to an mTBI.

CHAPTER NINE

Findings and Recommendations

While many service members in the MHS are diagnosed and treated for mTBI, little is known about their patterns of medical care. In 2013, there were more than 27,000 worldwide cases of TBI, and patients with mTBI represent 84 percent of all TBI cases among service members (DVBIC, 2014a). The sheer number of these injuries and the lack of information about how care is being provided pose significant challenges for the MHS. Further research is needed to understand more fully how care is delivered in the MHS and other settings (Manley and Maas, 2013). This report presents results from the first comprehensive study of the types and patterns of care delivered by the MHS to nondeployed active-duty service members who received an ICD-9 diagnosis for mTBI in 2012. This research was guided by six research questions corresponding to the Chapters Three through Eight:

1. How many nondeployed active-duty service members receive treatment for mTBI?
2. What are the characteristics of nondeployed active-duty service members who receive a diagnosis for mTBI in the MHS?
3. Where do service members with mTBI receive care?
4. What are the duration and patterns of care for service members in the six months after an mTBI diagnosis?
5. What kind of care do service members with mTBI receive?
6. Who receives persistent care?

To address these research questions, we examined health care utilization, in both the direct and purchased care systems, as along with other administrative data from the MHS. We identified all active-component service members who were diagnosed with a new mTBI in calendar year 2012. We then performed descriptive analyses on this cohort and examined their patterns of care, co-occurring diagnoses, treatment sources and settings, and diagnostic assessments. Our study is a first-ever effort to examine care provided to a census of patients in the MHS who have been diagnosed with an mTBI, offering a view of the landscape of care received through the MHS in the six months following the mTBI diagnosis. Using the ICD-9–based case definition we selected, we describe the characteristics of 16,378 service members who received a new mTBI diagnosis in 2012, the most recent calendar year for which we could examine subsequent care. We described the settings in which they received care, as well as the nature and duration of the care they received. Our approach provides an empirical foundation that can be used to guide future studies that use more detailed clinical data. In this chapter we describe our main findings and present considerations for policy and future research.

Summary of Findings

This report describes the cohort of nondeployed active-duty service members with a new mTBI diagnosis in 2012. Our findings are specific to the cohort that received care from the MHS in 2012, and this cohort represents the entire population of nondeployed active-duty service members (i.e., a census) diagnosed with an mTBI in year. That said, it would be reasonable to hypothesize that similarly drawn cohorts from the years since 2012 would result in similar findings. In other words, this view of the landscape of mTBI care may extend beyond 2012, but such hypotheses should be tested further in clinical and health systems studies.

Due to the nature of our data, we avoided inferring cause-and-effect relationships among variables, even when such an assumption would have seemed reasonable. For example, we did not attribute care received in the six months following the mTBI diagnosis to the mTBI itself, due to limitations in the way that ICD-9 codes are used for this injury. We acknowledge that a portion of the care received in those six months could have been for other conditions, such as extracranial trauma that occurred as a result of the incident that caused the mTBI. Our findings must be considered with this in mind.

Nondeployed Active-Duty Service Members with a New mTBI Tended to Be Young and Junior Enlisted

Among the 16,378 nondeployed active-duty service members who received treatment for a new mTBI diagnosis in 2012, 48 percent were between 18 and 24 years old, most (54 percent) were junior enlisted and had served in the military for an average of six years. Two-thirds had a history of deployment. The majority of the 2012 mTBI cohort were Army personnel (54 percent), with the other three services making up approximately equal proportions of the remainder of the cohort.

The age and service experience profile of the cohort could be explained in at least two ways. First, junior and more senior members of the military play different roles, with younger service members deploying at higher rates and serving in occupational specialties with greater risks of head injury (e.g., infantry). This is consistent with earlier research showing higher rates of mTBI among junior enlisted personnel (Cameron et al., 2012). Second, service members who are injured or ill, including those who have suffered an mTBI, may be unable to continue serving and may separate from the military sooner. However, members of the cohort who had a history of TBI (of any severity) at the time of their mTBI diagnosis, as well as those with persistent symptoms, were older than the general mTBI cohort, suggesting that the burden of TBI builds with military experience.

Many Nondeployed Active-Duty Service Members with a New mTBI Received Treatment for Co-Occurring Behavioral Health Conditions, Pain, and Sleep Disorders

We explored the rate at which the mTBI cohort received treatment for co-occurring behavioral health conditions, finding that 11–16 percent received treatment for each of the following conditions in the six months after the mTBI diagnosis: adjustment disorders, anxiety disorders, depression, alcohol abuse/dependence, and PTSD. Receipt of treatment for these conditions was more common among those who with a previous TBI diagnosis. We compared these rates in the six months before the 2012 mTBI diagnosis and in the six months after the diagnosis. For the five most commonly co-occurring behavioral health conditions, a larger percentage of the cohort received treatment after being diagnosed with an mTBI. For example, 12 percent of the cohort received treatment for depression after the mTBI diagnosis, compared to 8 percent before the diagnosis. One explanation might be that behavioral health conditions are identified through the patient's interaction with the health care system due to mTBI treatment, but the behavioral health condition may not be a consequence of the mTBI. Alternatively, the behavioral health condition could have developed as a consequence of the mTBI or as a psychiatric response to the same event that caused the brain injury. The data did not allow us to draw conclusions about the causality of these conditions, showing only that they co-occur with and are more frequent after an mTBI diagnosis.

We also explored treatment for nonbehavioral health conditions in the six months following the mTBI diagnosis, focusing particularly on the treatment of symptoms and conditions known to commonly or occasionally co-occur with an mTBI. Fifty-seven percent of the mTBI cohort received treatment for a non-headache pain condition, while 40 percent received treatment for headache and a quarter received treatment for a sleep disorder. As with behavioral health conditions, a higher proportion of the cohort received treatment in the six months after the mTBI diagnosis than did so in the six months before with mTBI diagnosis. Those with a history of TBI were more likely to receive treatment for these symptoms and conditions.

Most Nondeployed Active-Duty Service Members with a New mTBI Were Diagnosed in the Emergency Department and Received Follow-Up Treatment in Primary Care Settings

We found that 60 percent of the mTBI cohort was diagnosed in the direct care system, and, of these service members, 40 percent were diagnosed at a primary care clinic and 35 percent were diagnosed in an emergency department. Of the 40 percent who were diagnosed in the civilian purchased care network, the vast majority (80 percent) received their diagnosis in an emergency department. Taken together, this implies that half of all service members in the mTBI cohort were diagnosed in an emergency department. Service members with a history of TBI or deployment at the time of mTBI diagnosis were considerably less likely to be diagnosed in an emergency department than were those without this history.

On average, those in the 2012 mTBI cohort had their first health care encounter 17 days after the mTBI diagnosis, and 87 percent of these visits took place in the direct care system, with nearly half occurring in a primary care setting. Service members with a history of TBI or deployment were more likely to be treated for their follow-up visit in a behavioral health clinic, compared with those without TBI or deployment histories; those service members were more likely to be seen at a primary care clinic.

Most Nondeployed Active-Duty Service Members with mTBI Received Care for Only a Short Time After the mTBI Diagnosis, Suggesting a Quick Recovery

We found that most service members in the 2012 mTBI cohort received treatment for symptoms and conditions commonly or occasionally associated with mTBI for a month or less following their mTBI diagnosis. In fact, it appeared that service members received the largest portion of their care within the first week after diagnosis. Half to three-quarters of the mTBI cohort did not receive any treatment at all for behavioral health conditions or symptoms commonly or occasionally associated with mTBI. This suggests that, for the majority of service members with a new mTBI, recovery may be relatively quick. That said, 78 percent of the mTBI cohort had regular or frequent health care visits over the six months following their mTBI diagnosis, though it is likely that these visits were for conditions unrelated to the mTBI. A minority (10–20 percent) received treatment for three months or longer.

Nondeployed Active-Duty Service Members with a New mTBI Received a Variety of Diagnostic Assessments and Treatments, with Differences in Care by TBI History

The most common diagnostic assessments in the six months following an mTBI diagnosis were CT scans (33 percent), psychiatric evaluations (29 percent), and physical therapy evaluations (25 percent), though these assessments could have been for conditions other than the mTBI. Service members who had a history of TBI at the time of diagnosis were more likely to receive a wide range of diagnostic assessments, which may be explained by a need for more recovery time and more treatment.

We observed that psychotherapy and physical therapy were the most common treatments in the six months following the mTBI diagnosis, and they were received by 25–30 percent of the mTBI cohort. As with diagnostic assessments, members of the cohort who had a history of TBI at the time of diagnosis were more likely to receive many common treatments.

Although we were not able to determine whether service members filled prescriptions for medications associated with the mTBI or for another reason, we found that 62 percent of the cohort filled a prescription for analgesics in the six months following diagnosis. Opioids were also commonly filled (by half of the cohort), as were antidepressants (one-quarter of the cohort). A higher proportion of service members filled prescriptions for each of the medications we assessed in the six months following the mTBI diagnosis than in the six months before. Service members with a history of TBI at the time of mTBI diagnosis were more likely to fill most types of prescriptions than were those without a history of TBI.

A Minority of Nondeployed Active-Duty Service Members with mTBI Had Complex and Persistent Care Needs

We identified a subset of service members in the 2012 mTBI cohort who may have had ongoing care needs beyond the expected recovery period. Those with persistent care needs received treatment for co-occurring behavioral health problems and symptoms related to mTBI at a much higher rate than those without persistent problems. This group also used substantially more health services. Adjusted relative risk analysis indicated that previous TBI diagnoses and a history of deployment were predictive of receiving persistent care.

Less than a third of service members in the mTBI cohort who received treatment for PCS had a TBI diagnosis of any severity in the previous six months, indicating they may have been receiving treatment for an older injury or one that had never been diagnosed. Service members with a PCS diagnosis were also likely to experience behavioral health problems, as well as symptoms and conditions commonly or occasionally associated with mTBI, such as headache or sleep problems. It is important to remember, however, that our data documented only the co-occurrence of conditions; we were unable to directly link mTBI to these co-occurring conditions.

Limitations and Considerations for Future Analysis

Administrative data from the MHS hold significant promise for future studies of care patterns. These data are already collected for administrative purposes, can be examined longitudinally, and contain information on a census of patients. They are also inexpensive when compared with the cost of collecting clinical data in registries or through prospective clinical research.

Using already collected, deidentified data presents lower risks of disclosing protected health information and, therefore, lower risks to patients.

However, administrative data also present a number of limitations for studies of care patterns. A large proportion of data from administrative sources may be missing. Reliability of coding is also an issue. Data quality and lack of depth are particular concerns; key clinical information, explicit connections within a condition but across visits, and other important details are not available in data sets of this kind. These challenges largely arise from the fact that the data were collected for administrative and not research purposes. Throughout this report, we discussed a number of uncertainties that arise from these concerns. These uncertainties included specification of the cohort and attribution of care to an episode.

These limitations play out in specific ways for analyses of care in the MHS setting. In the course of our work, we encountered a lack of consensus about case definitions for mTBI and found evidence of inconsistent coding practices and confusing coding guidelines for clinical settings. In the following sections, we describe these findings in more detail.

Prevalence Estimates for mTBI Are Highly Sensitive to Case Definitions
Estimates of TBI are extremely sensitive to case definitions (AFHSC, 2009), and various definitions have been suggested for identifying TBI using ICD-9 diagnoses. These definitions come from civilian, military, and non-DoD government agencies or the academic literature and include classifications that go beyond the typical severity scale. While some of this variation is warranted to meet a variety of needs, it makes it more challenging to interpret surveillance and research. This is seen, for example, in the widely ranging estimates across studies (Carlson et al., 2011).

One area that should be a priority is identifying service members with ongoing treatment needs, which will require approaches that follow patients over time to characterize the life course of TBI and mTBI (see, e.g., Kristman et al., 2014, and Laborde, 2000; for a similar sentiment regarding research in the civilian sector, see Manley and Maas, 2013). Future work on case definitions and coding guidance should reflect who is at risk for or experiencing long-term or delayed presentations of mTBI as a means of predicting what types of care they may require. While most individuals with ongoing problems should receive a PCS diagnosis, this does not appear to be the case in practice, and questions have been raised about the validity of this diagnosis (Lagarde et al., 2014).

An important milestone will be the transition to ICD-10, Clinical Modification, which is discussed more in Appendix C. Currently, there are no government recommendations for coding mTBI using the ICD-10, though some may be forthcoming (see Appendix C). The ICD-10 differs fairly substantially from ICD-9, providing an opportunity to revisit the codes used to classify and identify mTBI. Likewise, the coding guidance could also be revised to make it more consistent with likely provider practice, as discussed next.

Providers, Within and Across Health Care Systems, Are Challenged by Distinct and Evolving Coding Guidance
Providers who cross between civilian and military health care systems may find very different guidance for coding an mTBI. Even within the MHS, coding guidance has evolved considerably over the past 15 years. The lack of clarity that characterizes the condition itself (see, e.g., Hyatt, Davis, and Barroso, 2014) is also expressed administratively through a combination of ambiguous codes (e.g., head injury, unspecified) and specialty codes that are not shared with

other conditions (e.g., history of TBI). The lack of uniform coding guidance is likely reflected in variation in coding practices (Helmick et al., 2012; Hoge, McGurk, et al., 2008; Kristman et al., 2014; Roozenbeek, Maas, and Menon, 2013).

Health Care Providers Use Inconsistent Coding Practices

For administrative codes to be applied consistently, there must be a shared understanding of how the codes are supposed to be applied. This can be achieved through awareness of current coding guidance put forward by DVBIC (using ICD-9 and ICD-10 diagnostic codes). While current TBI coding guidance stipulates that the TBI diagnosis itself should be used only for the initial visit and not subsequent visits, ICD-9 coding practice for most other conditions requires that the condition diagnosis be used for all visits (AFHSC, 2012; DoD, 2010). The changes in coding guidance and lack of clarity for providers who cross health care systems are real challenges for the consistency of mTBI coding practices.

Outcomes Data Are an Indispensable Resource for Future Research

Clinical outcomes, while largely outside the clinical, financial, and legal purposes of administrative data, are critically important for surveillance, research, and quality improvement efforts. However, there is little opportunity to examine the clinical outcomes of service members treated by the MHS. A means of tracking patients through possibly multiple care systems, over time, with standardized documentation, and past the episode of care, would vastly improve the value of these data. Extending outcomes to consider both clinical and nonclinical outcomes, such as patient experience and coordination of care,[1] social role participation, and perceived health-related quality of life, would provide a more complete picture of care quality (see, e.g., Wilde et al., 2010; Bombardier et al., 2010). Many types of outcome data, such as patient experience, are better gathered through surveys or other methods, rather than through administrative data.

Recommendations

1. Improve ICD-9 Coding Practices and Reconsider Current TBI Coding Guidance

Good administrative data should be considered integral to health care quality because these data help track the status of patients and the treatments and procedures they receive. DoD TBI coding guidance requires that providers record a TBI diagnosis only at the first visit, with subsequent visits coded with relevant symptom diagnostic codes. This coding guidance is different from that for any other condition and could be confusing to providers. Furthermore, the outcome from coding health care encounters in this way is that it is not possible to use administrative data to observe treatment for mTBI over time. In this report, we examined treatment for symptoms and conditions that may be associated with mTBI, but we were not able to determine whether treatment for these conditions was related to the mTBI. DoD should consider whether the advantages of the current TBI coding guidance outweigh the disadvantages for understanding the nature of care delivered to service members with TBI.

In addition, while identifying the most appropriate mechanisms to improve the reliability and consistency of coding was outside the scope of this study, our analysis suggested that there

---

[1]   As is done through CAHPS (Consumer Assessment of Healthcare Providers and Services) in the civilian sector.

may be variations in ICD-9 coding practices across the MHS. Future efforts should consider the facilitators and barriers to accurate coding for TBI treatment in the MHS, including practice setting and provider or coder characteristics.

2. Improve Data Quality to Increase Capacity for Research

The very nature and purpose of administrative codes pose real challenges for using them in research. Administrative codes are collected for multiple uses, including legal and financial reviews, that are largely unrelated to surveillance and research. This limits the data's utility for the purposes of analysis. Improving the connectivity between administrative claims and other clinical data (e.g., chart data, pharmacy data) can enhance their value and suggests the need for a more comprehensive method for obtaining data.[2] The current lack of connectivity limits the use of the data for clinically relevant research. For example, it is often difficult to determine, using administrative data, whether referrals were followed up on or whether a prescription that was ordered was filled. Creating more interoperable data streams will facilitate a wide range of research.

3. Identify Opportunities to Coordinate Care

Our results demonstrate that service members diagnosed with mTBI receive treatment in a wide variety of clinical settings. While not unique to mTBI, the specific challenges faced by these service members (and their providers) highlight the need to emphasize coordination of care and communication across providers, especially across direct- and purchased-care settings. First, it will be important to understand current challenges and strategies for coordinating mTBI care across the MHS and to then identify best practices and innovative mechanisms for care coordination. Broader health system changes, such as the introduction of patient-centered medical homes (AHRQ, 2012), may provide opportunities for coordination across a diverse set of providers. Another approach could be to enhance the role of the DVBIC Recovery Support System program or similar programs. DVBIC recovery support specialists may be an effective means of enhancing coordination across providers, settings, and systems (Martin et al., 2013).

4. Assess the Quality of Care for Service Members with mTBI

The data presented here are a first step toward assessing the quality of mTBI care by providing a baseline description of the service member population with mTBI and the care they receive. That said, the results are limited to the most obvious (and albeit most important) variables, are largely descriptive in nature, and raise as many questions as they answer. Future efforts need to extend these findings to examine not only the type of care that these service members receive but also the quality. Unfortunately, there are challenges in taking this next step.

The most notable challenge is the lack of validated quality measures for mTBI treatment, and future efforts will clearly need to develop such measures. Developing quality measures for mTBI will be challenging, however, given that there is great variation in the initial presentation and trajectory of mTBI across patients, and there are common comorbid conditions with similar presentations (most notably PTSD). There has been debate over whether the concept of an "average patient" is useful in this context, given the diversity of symptom presentation such that a simple standard of care against which to measure quality may be too general or impos-

---

[2] For example, through a database that spans the services and captures the continuum of care.

sible. This should not, however, stand in the way of developing clear guidelines around specific aspects of care, such as the appropriate use of pharmacotherapy in this population.

5. Extend These Results with Hypothesis-Driven, Multivariate Analyses

As noted earlier, this study was designed to establish a descriptive foundation for subsequent, hypothesis-directed studies. To that end, we identified a number of areas that should be explored with further multivariate analyses. In particular, this study provides the basis for a series of hypotheses about the relationships among patient, clinician, and setting factors in care patterns and outcomes among service members with mTBI. While this report identified a number of potential relationships among these variables, an exploration of why we observed certain differences and how best to address them was beyond the scope of this project. Multivariate analysis can take multiple variables into account, helping to clarify when observed differences may be due to other factors.

Examine Co-Occurring Conditions and Symptoms

Several co-occurring clinical conditions identified in our cohort should be considered for further examination. Tables 4.6 and 4.7 in Chapter Four shed an initial, descriptive light on what might be gained from such an approach, and there were interesting patterns in treatment for behavioral health conditions and conditions and symptoms commonly or occasionally co-occurring with mTBI. An extension of this research could involve factor analysis, cluster analysis, or other approaches that expand the scope from considering pairs of variables to considering multiple variables. If such clusters of conditions or symptoms could be identified and account for a substantial portion of the variation in the original data, then these clusters might be useful for subsequent analyses, such as those regarding episodes of care. For example, it may be the case that patients who experience a certain set of symptoms are more likely to need persistent care. Such an analysis would be complex, requiring substantial thought and care in conceptualizing these dependencies. It would likely require a novel conceptual model to rule out many contingencies and alternative explanations.

Explore Predictors of Care Patterns

Characterizing the course of care is a critical step in building statistical approaches to predicting it. The concept of a care episode, as used in this report, is one such approach, but specific inquiries could also examine particular aspects of the course of care, such as whether patients received specific types of care, whether they saw specific specialists, where they received care, and how treatment concluded.

In other words, it is important to identify predictors of the *patterns* of mTBI care. For example, does the course of care differ by diagnostic setting? Does the course of care differ for those who receive care from a TBI clinic? To what extent do variations in care patterns reflect differences in the initial severity of an mTBI?

Explore Variation in Care

Our results offer some evidence of variation in care by service and history of TBI, and it is important to understand the reasons for these variations. First, variations in care could reflect actual differences in the populations being seen. MTFs and their providers could be appropriately adjusting their approaches to diagnosis and treatment based on the unique needs of individual service members. Alternatively, there could be variability in diagnosis and treatment across providers due to differences in training and experience. These variations could be associated with a poorer quality of care. Clinical practice guidelines are designed to decrease inappropriate variability in providing care, thus ensuring that a service member will receive appropriate, high-quality care regardless of where he or she is seen. Understanding the reasons for observed differences can inform quality improvement initiatives and reduce inappropriate variations in care.

Future research in this area should leverage natural sources of clinical care variation. An examination of care received at MTFs of varying size and resources that accounts for the types of patients they treat could help shed light on one potential source of variation.

Examine a Clinical Cohort with Persistent mTBI-Related Problems

Our examination of a large population of service members showed that individuals with mTBI have persistent care needs. Improved understanding of this group is required to address these needs. As a first step, it will be important to accurately identify service members who have ongoing care needs and to determine the risk factors associated with persistent care. While administrative data allowed us to examine persistent care among the population of service members with mTBI, there are the limitations to this approach—most notably issues associated with proper diagnostic coding. Other data sources, such as clinical data or medical record data, would help in better identifying service members with long-term needs.

Clinical research could help determine the role of deployment and previous TBIs in the need for persistent care. While it is clear in our data that both of these variables are associated with persistent care, it is unclear whether these are causal factors. A better understanding of mediating variables that may contribute to continued health-seeking behavior would be needed for such a study. In the absence of experimental or quasi-experimental data, observational analysis of predefined subgroups would be useful.

Clinical research is also needed to detect whether persistent care patients are sicker overall or whether they are using more care as a result of the mTBI. This would allow us to measure the impact of clinical interventions on symptom persistence, identify inappropriate utilization, and test interventions to reduce symptom persistence.

Final Thoughts

As a signature injury of modern warfare, TBI affects more service members than ever before. Mild TBI, the most common TBI severity, can be challenging to identify and treat due to variations in symptom presentation and other factors. To deliver the most efficient and effective treatment for service members with an mTBI, it is important to first understand how many and which service members receive an mTBI diagnosis, where they receive care, the types of treatment they receive, and for how long they receive care. As we have highlighted throughout this report, the ultimate goal of improving quality of care (and subsequent clinical outcomes) depends on a solid evidence base. This report provides a first descriptive step in establishing that base by describing the population of nondeployed active-duty service members seeking care for an mTBI diagnosis in 2012, their clinical characteristics, and the care that they received.

Using ICD-9 Codes to Identify mTBI

Identification and tracking of mTBI patients are critical tasks when using claims data to study mTBI. In this study, we were able to assess health care utilization across the complete TRICARE system. This has some real advantages over other methods (e.g., survey, observation) in terms of power and generalizability. While administrative data have limitations (Hunt et al., 1999; Wynn et al., 2001; Birman-Deych et al., 2005), the use of these data enabled us to observe patients and treatments at near-population levels. In this appendix, we discuss the complexities of using administrative data to identify mTBI patients and the limitations that this imposed on our study.

As summarized in Table A.1, there are three critical stages that can pose challenges to patient identification and tracking: (1) presentation, (2) diagnosis/assessment, and (3) patient codes.

Those with mTBI Do Not Always Present for Care

Many studies assess patient populations, and because of that, estimates rely on *presentation for treatment*. While focusing on patients does not cause problems for the study methodology itself (i.e., internal validity), the study may be systematically excluding individuals who

Table A.1
Key Data Challenges and Validity for TBI

Critical Stage	Data Challenge	Validity Discussion
Presentation	When individuals with symptoms do not present to the health care system for diagnosis and treatment	This is a concern for external validity with regard to prevalence in the target population. In this study, looking at the landscape of care actually provided (i.e., not prevalence), it is not a validity concern except to note that there is a substantial TBI population *not* receiving care.
Diagnosis	When the clinical diagnosis made by health care professionals is incorrect, which could reflect inaccurate inclusion or exclusion in the mTBI population	The base rate of the non-mTBI population is much larger than the mTBI population, so the effect of inaccurate diagnosis is to dilute the mTBI population disproportionately. This creates a conservative bias in the treatment population. (It is important to note that this study did not make any direct comparisons between mTBI and non-mTBI populations.)
Coding	When administrative (e.g., ICD-9) codes do not reflect the clinical diagnoses	There are multiple potential coding challenges. For the definition of the study population, the reliability of coding likely poses the largest challenges.

reach diagnostic or exposure thresholds in the population but do not present for treatment (Roozenbeek, Maas, and Menon, 2013). Thus, the results of the study cannot address that part of the population.

Those Who Present for Care Do Not Always Receive a Correct Diagnosis

The second consideration for mTBI estimates is whether the patient has received a *correct diagnosis* after presenting for treatment (Peabody et al., 2004). Incorrect diagnoses can, of course, occur in both directions (i.e., patients can be incorrectly coded as having or not having an mTBI). This is especially challenging with mild TBI, for which diagnosis relies heavily on patient self-reports, and findings from diagnostic testing and symptomology may neither confirm nor disprove the existence of the condition (Brenner, Vanderploeg, and Terrio, 2009).

Patients with an mTBI Diagnosis May Not Receive Accurate Administrative Codes

Finally, if patients are identified or followed using administrative codes, it is critical to know whether the *coding accurately reflects diagnoses or symptoms* (Powell et al., 2008). Administrative coding is done for a diverse set of purposes, including financial and legal reasons. It is important to remember that the codes used to track patients and care at the population level reflect only part of a complex landscape of coding incentives. Further, coding is not always performed by the health care provider who attended the clinical consultation (Peabody et al., 2004). These and other reasons lead to additional considerations for their use. Patient record data (i.e., the patient's chart) are not included here because, at present, they are not always electronically accessible or searchable in the manner needed for this type of research. The following are some of the key challenges in interpreting codes related to mTBI:

- *Interrater reliability:* Were the codes applied consistently and appropriately across health care providers? If different providers use the codes in different ways, this affects the quality of the data. An associated challenge here is test-retest reliability: Is the application of codes consistent over time? Note that this is especially important in a field with changing coding guidance.
- *Content validity:* Do the codes represent a different construct from the diagnoses? This could relate to a difference in intended purpose.
- *Predictive validity:* Are the codes associated with mTBI symptoms good predictors for mTBI? (Note that this may not remain an issue with the transition to ICD-10 coding.)

Nosologists and our own experience suggest that codes are often inconsistent with mTBI coding guidance (Powell et al., 2008; Shore et al., 2005), which was a validity challenge for this study. However, the largest single challenge in this study was likely the reliability of the administrative coding. Providers and other health care administrative staff are quite variable in their coding practices. This is compounded in the case of mTBI, which is treated by a number of provider types and in a variety of settings. Coding guidance regarding TBI has also evolved (especially over the past decade), which may reduce reliability over time. To address these challenges, our approach focused primarily on a well-established and broad definition of mTBI, which casts a wide net on the mTBI population. In Appendix B, we present robustness analyses of the definition itself, using selected results to identify the impact of coding modification on results.

Table A.2, adapted from Bazarian et al. (2006) gives an overview of some of the strengths and limitations of using ICD-9 codes to identify patients with mTBI. Bazarian et al.'s analysis suggests that administrative codes are better at *ruling out* mTBI (reflected in their negative predictive value) than ruling it *in* (positive predictive value).[1] Generally, administrative data have better positive predictive values for more severe cases of TBI than for mild ones. Mild cases have less clear presentation and are also associated with many potential combinations of codes. Further, ambiguous but convenient codes, such as 959.01 (head injury, unspecified) tend to classify individuals into less severe categories of mTBI (Shore et al., 2005). Once a patient has presented and the treatment has been coded, those codes are significantly more likely to yield false positives than false negatives (i.e., overreporting). The ability of administrative codes to rule out mTBI at that point is quite successful (see Table A.2).

Comparatively, the DoD administrative case definition is designed to cast a wide net on mTBI. In effect, the DoD definition intentionally permits the inclusion of false positives to catch as many "true positives" as possible, which heightens the underlying permissiveness of the codes.

The challenge posed by the lower positive predictive value of the mTBI diagnostic codes offers different opportunities. It is important to note that Bazarian et al.'s 2006 study was conducted prior to the development and revisions to the DoD coding guidance and that their study does not use this definition. However, we suspect that these findings largely apply. Generally, the false positives (when there are so few false negatives) give the data a conservative bias, suggesting that the "treatment" group is made weaker, so we would be more confident in findings. For the purposes of this study, the introduction of probable non-mTBIs creates a more complicated landscape. First, we are not drawing comparisons between mTBI and non-mTBI cases, making testing less relevant to our analyses. Moreover, some mTBI patients may have been incorrectly *diagnosed*; however, this is likely to apply to a minority of cases. More likely,

Table A.2
Accuracy of ICD-9 Versus Clinical Diagnoses for mTBI

Characteristic	Point Estimate	95% Confidence Interval
Sensitivity	0.46	0.41–0.50
Specificity	0.98	0.98–0.98
Positive predictive value	0.24	0.21–0.26
Negative predictive value	0.99	0.99–0.99

SOURCE: Adapted from Bazarian, 2006, p. 34, Table 2.

---

[1] The positive predictive value is the number of true positive cases divided by the number of positive cases, including true positive cases and false positive cases. Similarly, the negative predictive value is the number of true negative cases divided by the number of negative cases, including true negative cases and false negative cases.

these are cases in which the codes represent inaccuracies or challenges in translating clinical—particularly complex clinical—information into administrative codes (MacIntyre, Ackland, and Chandraraj, 1997). This appears to be most challenging with mTBI when multiple injuries are present (Bazarian et al., 2006).

Comparison and Variation Using the Project and Other ICD-9 Definitions

Detailed Specifications of ICD-9 Project Definitions with Descriptions

Table B.1 lists the full ICD-9, Clinical Modification, codes in the DoD case definition used for this project. It includes the set of codes that formed the project's new case definition, with the code number, description, and any notation about loss of consciousness, as relevant.

Table B.1
Project New Case Definition, with Code Descriptions

ICD-9 Code	Description	
	Intracranial Injury	Loss of Consciousness
850: Concussion		
850.0		None
850.11		Brief, 30 minutes or less
850.5		Unspecified duration
850.9		Unspecified concussion
800.0: Closed fracture of vault of skull		
800.00	Without mention of intracranial injury	Unspecified state of consciousness
800.01	Without mention of intracranial injury	None
800.02	Without mention of intracranial injury	Brief, 59 minutes or less
800.06	Without mention of intracranial injury	Unspecified duration
800.09	Without mention of intracranial injury	Unspecified concussion
800.5: Open fracture of vault of skull		
800.50	Without mention of intracranial injury	Unspecified state of consciousness
800.51	Without mention of intracranial injury	None
800.52	Without mention of intracranial injury	Brief, 59 minutes or less
801.0: Closed fracture of base of skull		
801.00	Without mention of intracranial injury	Unspecified state of consciousness
801.01	Without mention of intracranial injury	None
801.02	Without mention of intracranial injury	Brief, 59 minutes or less

Table B.1— Continued

ICD-9 Code	Description	
	Intracranial Injury	Loss of Consciousness
801.0: Closed fracture of base of skull (cont.)		
801.06	Without mention of intracranial injury	Unspecified duration
801.09	Without mention of intracranial injury	Unspecified concussion
801.5: Open fracture of base of skull		
801.50	Without mention of intracranial injury	Unspecified state of consciousness
801.51	Without mention of intracranial injury	None
801.52	Without mention of intracranial injury	Brief, 59 minutes or less
803.0: Other closed skull fracture		
803.00	Without mention of intracranial injury	Unspecified state of consciousness
803.01	Without mention of intracranial injury	None
803.02	Without mention of intracranial injury	Brief, 59 minutes or less
803.06	Without mention of intracranial injury	Unspecified duration
803.09	Without mention of intracranial injury	Unspecified concussion
803.5: Other open skull fracture		
803.50	Without mention of intracranial injury	Unspecified state of consciousness
803.51	Without mention of intracranial injury	None
803.52	Without mention of intracranial injury	Brief, 59 minutes or less
804.0: Closed fractures involving skull or face with other bones		
804.00	Without mention of intracranial injury	Unspecified state of consciousness
804.01	Without mention of intracranial injury	None
804.02	Without mention of intracranial injury	Brief, 59 minutes or less
804.06	Without mention of intracranial injury	Unspecified duration
804.09	Without mention of intracranial injury	Unspecified concussion
804.5: Open fractures involving skull or face with other bones		
804.50	Without mention of intracranial injury	Unspecified state of consciousness
804.51	Without mention of intracranial injury	None
804.52	Without mention of intracranial injury	Brief, 59 minutes or less
950 and 959: Other head injuries		
959.01	Head injury, unspecified	NA

Relationships Between Codes and Code Subsets

In this section, we provide an overview of the relationships between subsets of codes in the project definition, specific codes of interest, and sets of codes representing other levels of TBI severity (as shown in Table B.2). For a selected number of these relationships, we highlight some key areas of interest for interpreting study results and for the TBI literature as a whole. These data reflect 2012 figures and draw from both active-duty and activated National Guard and reserve forces; thus, totals are larger than in the findings presented in the body of this report.

Concussion Codes

Sixty percent (13,992 of 23,354) of the new case definition could be identified with a concussion code. Among service members with a concussion diagnosis, there was relatively little overlap with skull fractures (only 1.2 percent). On the other hand, 41.7 percent of those with a concussion diagnosis also had a TBI history code on file. A smaller percentage of those with concussion were diagnosed and coded with PCS (10.4 percent) and late effects (12.8 percent). TBI, unclassified, had a very similar profile to the concussion codes but had a somewhat higher distribution of co-occurring codes later: PCS (25.6 percent), history of TBI (73.9 percent), and late effects (36.1 percent).

Head Injury, Unspecified (959.01)

This code was included as a provisional code in the guidance in 2003 CDC report to Congress (National Center for Injury Prevention and Control, 2003). It also receives some discussion elsewhere in the literature (see, e.g., Shore, 2005) due to concerns about its lack of diagnostic distinctiveness. It is unclear whether the code will remain in future civilian or military coding guidance under the ICD-10, Clinical Modification. For service members with a 959.01 code, we see that 24.7 percent had a co-occurring concussion diagnosis, and 26.4 percent had a co-occurring concussion or skull fracture diagnosis. Notably, the 959.01 code *alone* would identify 37.7 percent (8,800) of the new mTBI population, using the project's definition (data not shown in Table B.2).

History of TBI, V-Code (V15.52)

V-codes represented a very large group within the coded population. In 2012, there were 36,718 uses of the history of TBI v-code (any severity), compared with 13,992 codings for mild concussions and 27,584 service members who would have been categorized into the new mTBI population *or* post-concussion group. The v-codes had roughly the same co-occurrence with new mTBI codes (19.1 percent) as with late-effect codes (20.1 percent).

Late Effects

Late-effects codes (905.0, 907.0) co-occurred intensively with a history of TBI code (V15.52). Of those with a V15.52 code, nearly 94 percent also carried a late-effect code. Of those with a late-effect code, 28.2 percent had a diagnostic code for a new mTBI, and 19.8 percent had a concussion code.

Table B.2
Relationships Between ICD-9 Codes and Codes in the Project Data

Diagnosis	Number	TBI, Mild (just concussions)	TBI, Mild (just skull fractures)	TBI, Mild (concussions + skull fractures)	Head Injury, Unspecified (959.01)	TBI, Mild (concussions + skull fractures + 959.01)	TBI, Mild (concussions + skull fractures + 959.01 + PCS)	TBI, Moderate	TBI, Severe	TBI, Penetrating	TBI, Unclassified	Post-Concussion	TBI History (V15.52)	Late Effects
						% of 2012 mTBI Cohort with Code								
TBI mild (just concussions)	13,992	—	1.2	100.0	21.1	100.0	100.0	4.1	0.3	0.1	9.4	10.4	41.7	12.8
TBI mild (just skull fractures)	734	23.4	—	100.0	38.3	100.0	100.0	32.4	3.8	5.6	21.4	7.8	32.6	19.9
TBI mild (concussions + skull fractures)	14,554	96.1	5.0	—	21.6	100.0	100.0	5.0	0.4	0.4	9.7	10.2	41.1	12.9
Head injury, unspecified (959.01)	11,949	24.7	2.4	26.4	—	100.0	100.0	5.2	0.6	0.4	5.7	7.0	15.4	5.1
TBI, mild (concussions + skull fractures + 959.01)	23,354	59.9	3.1	62.3	51.2	—	100.0	4.3	0.4	0.3	7.6	8.1	30.0	9.5
TBI, mild (concussions + skull fractures + 959.01 + PCS)	27,584	50.7	2.7	52.8	43.3	84.7	—	3.9	0.3	0.3	10.0	22.2	34.6	12.0
TBI, moderate	1,615	35.2	14.7	45.4	38.1	61.7	65.8	—	5.2	4.7	33.0	13.8	48.1	25.9
TBI, severe	136	31.6	20.6	45.6	49.3	67.6	69.9	61.8	—	12.5	57.4	11.0	52.9	41.2
TBI, penetrating	133	12.8	30.8	39.9	36.1	50.4	54.1	57.1	12.8	—	51.1	9.8	51.9	37.6
TBI, unclassified	5,557	23.6	2.8	25.5	12.4	31.7	49.5	9.6	1.4	1.2	—	25.6	73.9	36.1
Post-concussion	6,112	23.8	0.9	24.3	13.8	30.8	100.0	3.6	0.2	0.2	23.3	—	58.3	25.4
TBI history (V15.52)	36,718	15.9	0.7	16.3	5.0	19.1	26.0	2.1	0.2	0.2	11.2	9.7	—	20.1
Late effects	7,846	22.8	1.9	24.0	7.8	28.2	42.3	5.3	0.7	0.6	25.6	19.8	93.8	—

NOTE: Percentages are calculated within the rows.

Comparison of Project Definition to Other Definitions

This study used the DoD definition of mTBI as the basis of identifying patients with the condition. Table B.3 shows the DoD definition and two other case definitions for mTBI based on ICD-9, Clinical Modification, codes: (1) the CDC's 2003 report to Congress and (2) a concussion-only definition, which included a small number of codes for identifying mTBI.

These definitions offer a breadth of conceptualization for mTBI, from the DoD definition, which casts a relatively wide net for thinking about mTBI in the military, to the CDC definition, which puts forward a conceptualization of mTBI for civilians, and the concussion-only definition, which offers a very narrow construct for mTBI centering strictly on concussion.

Table B.3
Study Definition Compared with Other mTBI Definitions

Diagnostic Category	DoD Definition	CDC, 2003 Definition	Concussion Only
850: Concussion	850.0 850.11 850.5 850.9	850.0 850.11 850.12 850.5 850.9	850.0 850.11
854: Intracranial injury		854.01 854.02 854.06 854.09	
800.0: Closed fracture of vault of skull	800.00 800.01 800.02 800.06 800.09	800.00 800.01 800.02 800.06 800.09	
800.5: Open fracture of vault of skull	800.50 800.51 800.52	800.50 800.51 800.52 800.56 800.59	
801.0: Closed fracture of base of skull	801.00 801.01 801.02 801.06 801.09	801.00 801.01 801.02 801.06 801.09	
801.5: Open fracture of base of skull	801.50 801.51 801.52	801.50 801.51 801.52 801.56 801.59	
803.0: Other closed skull fracture	803.00 803.01 803.02 803.06 803.09	803.00 803.01 803.02 803.06 803.09	
803.5: Other open skull fracture	803.50 803.51 803.52	803.50 803.51 803.52 803.56 803.59	

Table B.3— Continued

Diagnostic Category	DoD Definition	CDC, 2003 Definition	Concussion Only
804.0: Closed fractures involving skull or face with other bones	804.00 804.01 804.02 804.06 804.09	804.00 804.01 804.02 804.06 804.09	
804.5: Open fractures involving skull or face with other bones	804.50 804.51 804.52	804.50 804.51 804.52 804.56 804.59	
950 and 959: Other head injuries	959.01	959.01	
310: Post-concussion syndrome	310.2		
TBI history (current standard; 2010–present)	V15.52 (specific extenders for mTBI)		V15.52 (specific extenders for mTBI)

SOURCES: National Center for Injury Prevention and Control, 2003; DVBIC, 2013.

ICD-9 to ICD-10 Considerations

The U.S. Department of Health and Human Services issued a rule in 2009 for a single compliance date for ICD-10 implementation. The original implementation date was October 1, 2013, which was adopted by Defense Health Agency and was to apply throughout the TRICARE management system. Following two subsequent Department of Health and Human Services final rules, the current target implementation date was October 1, 2015.

The ICD-10 was developed in the 1980s but was not implemented in any capacity in the United States until the late 1990s. The U.S. version is the ICD-10, Clinical Modification. While there has been extensive work to define general TBI and mTBI populations using ICD-9 data, work using the ICD-10 is considerably less advanced, particularly for mTBI (Orman et al., 2012). However, revisions to the definitions over the past decade (e.g., history of injury codes), along with growing awareness of the sensitivity and specificity challenges associated with the administrative codes for TBI (Bazarian et al., 2006), suggest that the movement to the ICD-10 offers opportunities to create better case definitions and more streamlined coding guidance.

Some studies have attempted to characterize the TBI population using ICD-10 codes. Prior to the CDC's 2003 *Report to Congress on Mild Traumatic Brain Injury in the United States: Steps to Prevent a Serious Public Health Problem* (National Center for Injury Prevention and Control, 2003), in 2002, Marr and Coronado at the CDC submitted surveillance standards proposing mortality coding recommendation for TBI using ICD-10 (Marr and Coronado, 2004, research conducted in 2002; Orman et al., 2012), as shown in Table C.1. However, the recommendation was not included in the 2003 report to Congress.

We include this section as a guide at a time when many civilian practitioners are undergoing transitions to ICD-10 and DoD is on the cusp of transition. While it was not possible to include ICD-10 case definitions or data in our analysis, the tables in this appendix give readers some idea of how these two coding systems relate to each other during this transitional period and for future years.

In 2011, Chen and Colantonio conducted a review of studies internationally (i.e., not exclusive to the ICD-10) that classified TBI using ICD codes. In Table C.2, we aggregate some of their findings, highlighting TBI codes that were most often present. While not a quantitative result, it reflects some level of perceived expert utility in the coding constructs. However, we must note that while there is substantial overlap, not all of these codes are relevant to an ICD-10 construct.

At the time of this study, the CDC and its partners from the National Center on Health Statistics were preparing a proposed ICD-10, Clinical Modification, surveillance case definition for TBI. That work and subsequent research ensuring the reliability and validity of these administrative codes will be critical to future epidemiologic and research endeavors. As we

Table C.1
Recommended ICD-10 Codes for TBI Mortality, 2002

ICD-10 Code	Description
S01.0–S01.9	Open wound of the head
S02.0, S02.1, S02.3, S02.7–S02.9	Fracture of skull and facial bones
S04.0	Injury to optic nerve and pathways
S06.0–S06.9	Intracranial injury
S07.0, S07.1, S07.8, S07.9	Crushing injury of head
S09.7–S09.9	Other and unspecified injuries of head
T01.0	Open wounds involving head with neck
T02.0	Fractures involving head with neck
T04.0	Crushing injuries involving head with neck
T06.0	Injuries of brain and cranial nerve with injuries of nerves and spinal cord at neck
T90.1, T90.2, T90.4, T90.5, T90.8, T90.9	Sequelae of injuries of head

SOURCE: Compiled from Marr and Coronado, 2004.

highlight in this report, the guidance around coding (in conjunction with a coding schema) is also important. Providers and other personnel in the health care setting who are responsible for applying administrative codes must understand the codes, should not find conflicting and duplicative codes, and, most importantly, must not find the task of coding too burdensome. When these elements fail, as we have observed, codes are misapplied, and coders employ short-cuts or default to the path of least resistance. It is possible, of course try to change the provider, but altering the guidance is more likely to be successful.

Table C.2
Frequency of Use of ICD-10 Codes for Identifying TBI in the Literature

ICD-10 Code	Description	Number of Mentions
F07.2	Post-concussion syndrome	2
S00	Superficial injury of head	2
S01.0–S01.6	Open wound(s) of scalp, open wound of eyelid and periocular area, open wound of nose, open wound of ear, open wound of cheek and temporomandibular area, open wound of lip and oral cavity	5
S01.7–S01.9	Multiple open wounds of head, open wound of other parts of head, open wound of head, part unspecified	7
S02.0	Fracture of vault of skull	12
S02.1	Fracture of base of skull	12
S02.2	Fracture of nasal bones	6
S02.3	Fracture of orbital floor	10
S02.4	Fracture of malar and maxillary bones	6
S02.5	Fracture of tooth	6
S02.6	Fracture of mandible	6
S02.7	Multiple fractures involving skull and facial bones	12
S02.8	Fracture of other skull and facial bones	12
S02.9	Fracture of skull and facial bones, part unspecified	12
S03	Dislocation, sprain and strain of joints and ligaments of head	4
S04	Injury of cranial nerves	4
S04.0	Injury to optic nerve and pathways	6
S05	Injury of eye and orbit	3
S06	Intracranial Injuries	14
S06.0	Concussion	14
S06.2–S06.3	Diffuse brain injury, focal brain injury	14
S07.0	Crushing injury of face	8
S07.1	Crushing injury of skull	9
S07.8	Crushing injury to other parts of head	8
S07.9	Crushing injury of head, part unspecified	9
S08	Traumatic amputation of part of head	3
S09.0	Injury of blood vessels of head, not elsewhere classified	6
S09.1	Injury of muscle and tendon of head	6
S09.2	Traumatic rupture of ear drum	6
S09.7	Multiple, injuries of head	11
S09.8	Other specified injuries to the head	10

Table C.2— Continued

ICD-10 Code	Description	Number of Mentions
S09.9	Unspecified injuries to the head	11
T01.0	Open wounds involving head with neck	1
T02.0	Fractures involving head with neck	2
T04.0	Crushing injuries involving head with neck	3
T04.1–T04.9	Crushing injuries of head with neck	1
T06.0	Other injuries involving brain, cranial nerves, and spinal cord at neck level	2
T06.1–T06.9	Injuries of brain and cranial nerves	1
T90.1	Sequelae of open wound of head	2
T90.2	Sequelae of fracture of skull and facial bones	3
T90.3	Sequelae of cranial nerves	0
T90.4	Sequelae of fracture of eye and orbit	2
T90.5	Sequelae of intracranial injury	3
T90.8	Sequelae of other specified injuries to the head	3
T90.9	Sequelae of unspecified injuries of the head	3
T96	Sequelae of poisoning by drugs, medicaments and biological substances	1
T97	Sequelae of toxic effects of substances chiefly non-medicinal as to source	1
T98.2	Sequelae of certain early complications of trauma	1

SOURCE: Compiled from Chen and Colantonio, 2011.

Variable Definitions

Co-Occurring Conditions

We categorized co-occurring conditions using ICD-9 codes, as shown in Tables D.1 and D.2.

Table D.1
ICD-9 Codes for Behavioral Health Conditions

Condition	ICD-9 Codes
Adjustment disorders	309.0, 309.1, 309.23–24, 309.28–29, 390.3, 309.4, 309.82–83, 309.89, 309.9
Anxiety disorders	293.84, 300.00–02, 300.09, 300.20–23, 300.29, 300.3, 300.89, 300.9
Acute stress disorders	308.0–4, 308.9
Alcohol abuse/dependence	303.00–03, 303.90–93, 305.00–03
ADD/ADHD	314.00–01, 314.8–9
Bipolar disorder	296.00–05, 296.10, 296.14, 296.40–45, 296.50–55, 296.60–64, 296.7, 296.80–82, 296.89
Delirium/dementia	293.0–1, 294.0, 294.8–9, 301.0, 310.2, 310.89, 310.9
Depression	293.83, 296.20–26, 296.30–36, 300.4, 311
Drug abuse/dependence	304.00–03, 304.10–13, 304.20–23, 304.30–33, 304.40–43, 304.50, 304.53, 304.60–63, 304.70, 304.71–73, 304.80–83, 304.90–93, 305.20–23, 305.30, 305.32–33, 305.40–43, 305.50–53, 305.60–63, 305.70–73, 305.80–81, 305.90–93
Personality disorders	301.0, 301.10, 301.12–13, 301.20, 301.22, 301.3–4, 301.50–51, 301.59, 301.6–7, 301.81–83, 301.89, 301.9
PTSD	309.81

Table D.2
ICD-9 Codes for Symptoms and Conditions Commonly or Occasionally Co-Occurring with mTBI

Condition	ICD-9 Codes
Alteration in mental status	780.02, 780.97
Cognitive problems	799.51–55, 799.59, 780.93, 331.83
Communication disorders	784.3, 784.51, 784.59–61, 784.69
Dizziness/vertigo	386.00, 386.03, 386.10–12, 386.19, 386.2 , 386.30, 386.35, 386.40, 386.42–43, 386.50, 386.53, 386.58, 386.9, 780.4
Gait and coordination problems	781.2–3
Headache	339.10–12, 339.20–22, 339.3, 339.41–44, 339.82–85, 339.89, 339.00–03, 346.00–03, 346.10–13, 346.20–21, 346.30, 346.40, 346.51, 346.70–73, 346.80–82, 346.90–93, 784.0
Hearing problems	388.10–12, 388.2, 388.30–32, 388.40, 388.42–45, 388.5, 388.9, 389.00–06, 389.10–22, 398.8, 398.9
Non-headache pain	307.8, 307.89, 338–338.4, 355, 355.9, 356–356.9, 357.2, 357.9, 524.6, 710–733.99
Skin sensation disturbances	782.0
Sleep disorders and symptoms	307.40–49, 327.00–.02, 327.09–15, 327.19–24, 327.26–27, 327.29, 327.30–31, 327.33, 327.35–36, 327.39, 327.40–44, 327.49, 327.51, 327.53, 327.59, 327.8, 347.00–01, 347.10, 780.50–59
Smell and taste disturbances	781.1
Syncope and collapse	780.2
Vision problems	377.75, 377.9, 378.00–01, 378.05, 378.10–11, 378.15, 378.17, 378.20–24, 378.30–35, 378.40–43, 378.45, 378.50–55, 378.60, 379.50–52, 379.54, 379.56–58, 379.8, 379.90–93

Diagnostic Assessments and Therapies

We categorized diagnostic assessments and therapies using CPT codes as follows.

Imaging
- CT (70450, 70460, 70470, 70480, 70486, 70487, 70496)
- MRI (70540, 70543, 70544, 70547, 70549, 70551, 70552, 70553, 76498).

Assessments
- Electroencephalography (95812, 95813, 95816, 95819, 95950, 95951, 95953, 95957)
- Vestibular testing (92531–92534, 92540–92546, 92548)
- Evaluation of speech, language, voice, communication, or auditory processing (92506)
- Audiology examinations (92550–92700, except 92552 and 92559)
- Neuropsychological assessment (96118, 96119, 96120)
- Neurobehavioral status exam (96116)
- Sensorimotor examination (92060)

- Psychiatric diagnostic evaluation
  - 2012 (90801, 90802)
  - 2013 (90791)
- Health and behavior assessment (96150, 96151)
- Sleep studies (95805–95811)
- Physical therapy evaluation (97001, 97002)
- Occupational therapy evaluation (97003, 97004).

Therapies
- Individual psychotherapy
  - 2012 (90804–90815, 90845)
  - 2013 (90785, 90832, 90833, 90834, 90836, 90837, 90838, 90839)
- Group psychotherapy (90853, 90857)
- Family psychotherapy (90846, 90847, 90849)
- Cognitive rehabilitation (97532)
- Speech therapy (92506, 92507, 92508)
- Sensory integration therapy (97533)
- Health and behavior intervention (96152–96155)
- Physical therapy: therapeutic exercise, neuromuscular reeducation, and physical therapy activities (97110, 97112, 97530)
- CPAP/BiPAP (94660, E0470, E0471, E0601)
- Neuromuscular electrical stimulation (97014, 97032)
- Occupational therapy (97535, 97537, 97545)
- Complementary and alternative medicine (CAM)
  - Acupuncture (97810, 97811, 97813, 97814)
  - Biofeedback (90875, 90876, 90901, 90911)
  - Chiropractic (98940–98943)
  - Hypnotherapy (90880)
  - Massage (97124)
  - Osteopathic (98925–98929).

Medications

Table D.3 lists the medications included in each medication class in the study. We categorized all prescriptions filled by service members in the 2012 mTBI cohort by medication class and included in the analysis only those classes that were potentially relevant to mTBI.

Table D.3
Medications Included in Each Medication Class

Medication Class	Medications Included in Class
Alcohol/drug pharmacologic treatment	Antabuse, butorphanol tartrate, Butrans, Campral, disulfiram, naloxone, naltrexone, Narcan, Nubain, pentazocine-naloxone, Revia, Suboxone, Subutex, Vivitrol
Analgesics (NSAIDs, acetaminophen, and other)	Acephen, acetaminophen, acetaminophen-butalbital, Advil, analgesic, Anaprox, APAP, Arthrotec, aspirin, Aspir-Low, butalbital, Caldolor, Cambia, Cataflam, Celebrex, children's aspirin, children's ibuprofen, Children's Motrin, children's pain and fever, Children's Q-Pap, Children's Tylenol, Daypro, diclofenax, potassium, diclofenac sodium, diflunisal, Duexis, Ecotrin, Epidrin, Esgic, etodolac, Feldene, FeverAll, Fioricet, Fiorinal, Flector, flurbiprofen, Genepap, Genebs, ibuprofen, Icy Hot, Indocin, indomethacin, isomethept-dichloralp-acetamin, ketoprofen, ketorolac tromethamine, Mapap, meloxicam, Midrin, Migquin, Mobic, Motrin, muscle rub, nabumetone, Naprelan, naproxen, Ofirmev, Orbivan, oxaprozin, pain and fever, pain relief, extra strength pain reliever, pain reliever, pain relieving rub, Panalgesic, Pennsaid, Phrenilin Forte, piroxicam, Ponstel, Prodrin, Q-Pap, Relagesic, salsalate, Sprix, sulindac, Thera-Gesic, tolmetin sodium, Toradol, Tylenol, Tylenol Extra Strength, Vimovo, Voltaren, Zebutal
Anticonvulsants/mood stabilizers	carbamazepine, Depakote, divalproex, Epitol, gabapentin, Gralise, Horizant, Keppra, Lamictal, lamotrigine, levetiracetam, lithium, Lithobid, Lyrica, Mysoline, Neurontin, oxcarbazepine, primidone, Tegretol, Topamax, topiramate, Trileptal, valproate sodium, Vimpat, Zonegran, zonisamide
Antidepressants	amitriptyline, bupropion, Celexa, chlordiazepoxide-amitriptyline, citalopram, clomipramine, Cymbalta, desipramine, doxepin, Effexor, Elavil, escitalopram oxalate, fluoxetine, fluvoxamine maleate, imipramine, Lexapro, Luvox, mirtazapine, nefazodone, norpramin, nortriptyline, Pamelor, paroxetine, Paxil, perphenazine-amitriptyline, Pristiq, Prozac, Remeron, sertraline, Silenor, Sinequan, Tofranil, trazodone, venlafaxine, Viibryd, Vivactil, Wellbutrin, Zoloft, Zyban
Antipsychotics	Abilify, chlorpromazine, fluphenazine, Geodon, Haldol, haloperidol, Invega, Latuda, olanzapine, quetiapine, Risperdal, risperidone, Saphris, Seroquel, thioridazine, trifluoperazine, ziprasidone, Zyprexa
Benzodiazepines	alprazolam, Ativan, chlordiazepoxide, chlorazepate, Diastat AcuDial, diazepam, flurazepam, Halcion, lorazepam, midazolam, oxazepam, Restoril, temazepam, Tranxene, triazolam, Valium, Xanax
Headache medications	Frova, Imitrex, Maxalt, Relpax, rizatriptan, sumatriptan, Sumavel DosePro, Treximet, Zomig
Muscle relaxants	Amrix, baclofen, carisoprodol, chlorzoxazone, cyclobenzaprine, Dantrium, Flexeril, Lorzone, metaxalone, methocarbamol, Norflex, orphenadrine, Robaxin, Skelaxin, Soma, tizanidine, vecuronium bromide, Zanaflex
Opioids	acetaminophen-codeine, Ascomp with Codeine, Avinza, butalbital-caffeine-acetaminophen-codeine, butalbital compound with codeine, codeine sulfate, Demerol, Dilaudid, Duragesic, Duramorph, Endocet, Exalgo, fentanyl, fentanyl citrate, hydrocodone, hydromorphone, Kadian, Lortab, meperidine, methadone, morphine suflate, MS Contin, MSIR, Norco, Nucynta, Opana, oxycodone, Oxycontin, oxymorphone, Percocet, Primlev, Reprexain, Roxicet, Roxicodone, Rybix, Sublimaze, tramadol, Tylenol with Codeine 3, Tylox, Ultracet, Ultram, Vicodin, Vicoprofen
Sleep aids	Ambien, Atarax, Buspar, buspirone, chloral hydrate, hydroxyzine, Inapsine, Intermezzo, Lunesta, Rozerem, Sonata, Vistaril, zaleplon, zolpidem
Stimulants	Adderall, ammonia inhalant, amphetamine salt combo, Concerta, Dexedrine, dextroamphetamine sulfate, dextroamphetamine amphetamine, Focalin, Methylin, methylphenidate, modafinil, Nuvigil, Provigil, Ritalin, Vyvanse

Additional Analyses

In this appendix, we present several additional analyses regarding service members' mTBI diagnosis and treatment locations, TBI history, and deployment history:

- analyses by service, TBI history, and deployment history relative to location of diagnosis
- analyses by service, TBI history, and deployment history relative to location of next health care encounter
- analyses by service and deployment history relative to treatment for co-occurring conditions, receipt of diagnostic evaluations and assessments, receipt of therapies, and filled prescriptions.

Location of mTBI Diagnosis

Figures E.1–E.3 describe the location of initial diagnosis by service, whether the service member was observed to have a history of TBI, and whether the service member had a history of deployment at the time of mTBI diagnosis, respectively.

The results by service (Figure E.1) mirror the overall findings reported in Chapter Five: The initial diagnostic visit most commonly took place in an MTF in direct care settings or in emergency departments in both the direct and purchased care networks. However, Army personnel were much more likely to be diagnosed with mTBI in an MTF primary care clinic than other service members (34 percent versus 10 percent, $p < 0.0001$); Navy, Air Force, and Marine Corps personnel groups were more likely to receive their diagnosis in a civilian emergency department. Approximately one-fifth of Army, Navy, and Marine Corps personnel were diagnosed in direct care emergency departments, but the rate was lower for Air Force personnel (14 percent). Army and Marine Corps personnel were relatively more likely to be diagnosed in a direct care behavioral health or neurology setting ($p < 0.0001$).

Figure E.2 shows that service members who had a history of TBI were substantially less likely to be diagnosed in an emergency department than were individuals who did not have a history of TBI ($p < 0.0001$). The largest difference was among those who were diagnosed in the purchased care network, where one-fifth of patients with a history of TBI were diagnosed in a civilian emergency department, compared with one-third of service members without a history of TBI ($p < 0.0001$). This difference was offset in most other settings—most notably MTF primary care and neurology clinics, where service members with a history of TBI were more likely than those without a prior TBI to receive their initial diagnosis ($p < 0.0001$).

Figure E.1
Location of mTBI Diagnosis, by Service

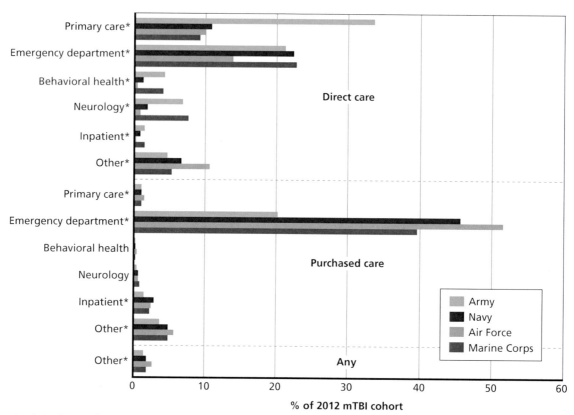

*Statistically significant difference at p < 0.0001.

RAND *RR844-E.1*

Figure E.2
Location of mTBI Diagnosis, by TBI History

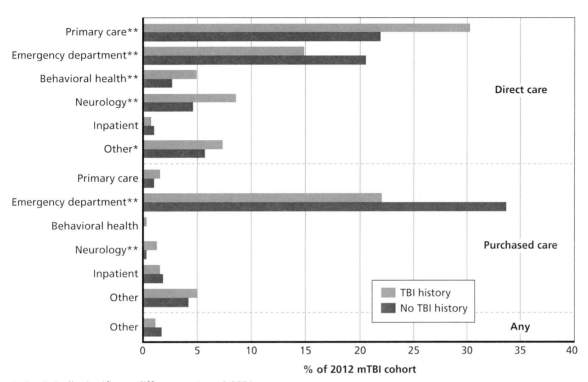

% of 2012 mTBI cohort

**Statistically significant difference at p < 0.0001.
*Statistically significant difference at p < 0.007.

RAND RR844-E.2

Figure E.3 shows the location of initial mTBI diagnosis according to whether the service member had a history of deployment as of the date of diagnosis. Like those with a history of TBI, service members who deployed prior to receiving an mTBI diagnosis were much more likely to be diagnosed in an MTF primary care clinic (p < 0.0001), whereas those who had no history of deployment were considerably more likely to be diagnosed in an emergency department (p < 0.0001). Those with a history of deployment were also more likely to be diagnosed in a direct care behavioral health or neurology setting (p < 0.0001).

Figure E.3
Location of mTBI Diagnosis, by Deployment History

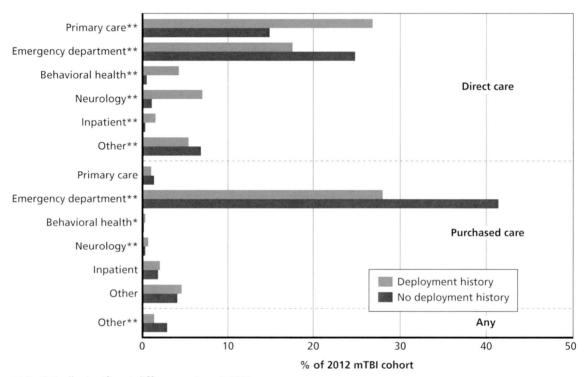

** Statistically significant difference at p < 0.0001.
 * Statistically significant difference at p ≤ 0.006.
RAND RR844-E.3

Location of First Health Care Encounter

As with the initial diagnosis, we considered whether there were differences across services and by history of TBI or deployment in the place of service for the first visit following diagnosis. Figures E.4–E.6 show these results.

Army and Air Force personnel were much more likely than Navy and Marine Corps personnel to have their first health care encounter in an MTF primary care clinic, by a difference of as much as 15 percentage points (p < 0.0001). On the other hand, they were noticeably less likely to visit other direct care settings for their follow-up visit. Army and Marine Corps personnel were relatively more likely to be seen in a direct care behavioral health clinic.

There were few differences in the setting of the first health care encounter between those who did and did not have a history of TBI at the time of the mTBI diagnosis. The vast majority of first health care encounters occurred in MTF primary care clinics or in settings we have categorized as "other" direct care (e.g., optometry, audiology, physical therapy). The only difference between these two groups was whether these health care encounters occurred in primary care or behavioral health settings. Members of the cohort with a history of TBI were more likely to have their first health care encounter in a behavioral health clinic than in a primary care clinic.

Figure E.4
Location of First Health Care Encounter, by Service

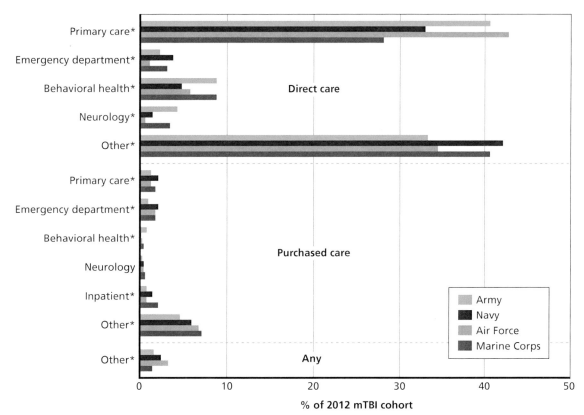

*Statistically significant difference at p < 0.0001.

RAND RR844-E.4

Figure E.5
Location of First Health Care Encounter, by TBI History

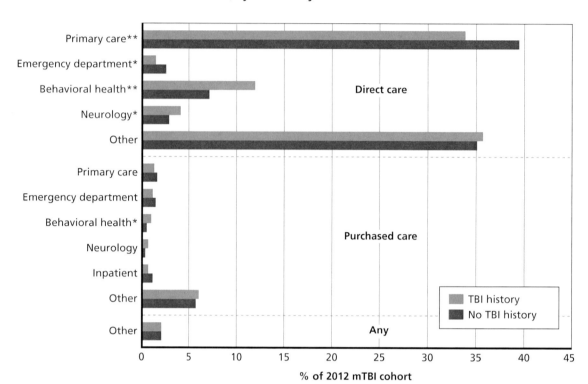

**Statistically significant difference at p < 0.001.
*Statistically significant difference at p < 0.05.
RAND *RR844-E.5*

The differences in the location of service members' first health care encounter by deployment history were also small (see Figure E.6). Service members who had a history of deployment at the time of the mTBI diagnosis were relatively more likely to have their first follow-up visit in a behavioral health setting than in a primary care clinic.

Figure E.6
Location of First Health Care Encounter, by Deployment History

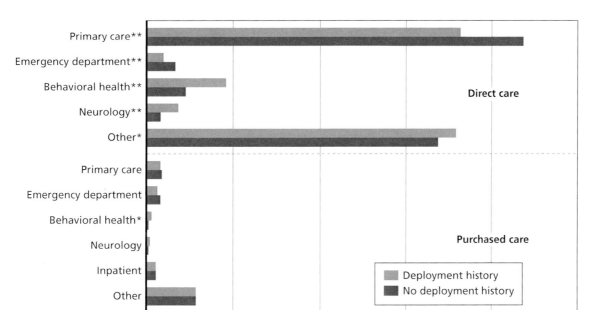

** Statistically significant difference at p < 0.0001.
 * Statistically significant difference at p < 0.01.
RAND *RR844-E.6*

Diagnostic Assessments, Treatments, and Medications, by Service and Deployment History

We explored treatment for co-occurring behavioral health conditions in the six months following the initial mTBI diagnosis by service branch. Figure E.7 shows, by service, receipt of treatment for co-occurring behavioral health diagnoses in the six months following the initial mTBI diagnosis. All differences by service branch were statistically significant (p < 0.0001) for all except delirium and dementia, for which differences were significant at p < 0.05. Army personnel were more likely to receive treatment for all behavioral health diagnoses except alcohol abuse/dependence and acute stress disorder, both of which were more common among Marine Corps personnel. Army and Marine Corps personnel were five times as likely as Navy and Air Force personnel to receive treatment for co-occurring PTSD, which may reflect greater exposure to direct combat than other branches.

Figure E.7
Treatment for Behavioral Health Conditions in the Six Months After mTBI Diagnosis, by Service

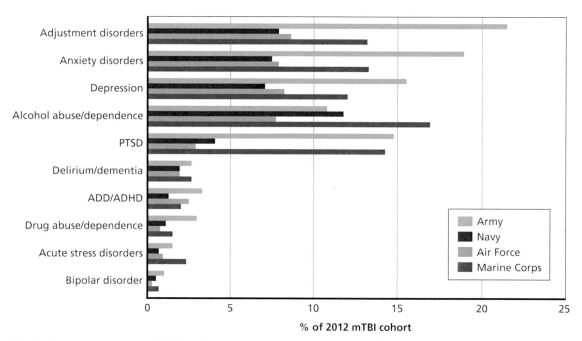

NOTE: With the exception of delirium/dementia (p < 0.05) treatment, all differences were significant at p < 0.0001.
RAND *RR844-E.7*

Figure E.8 shows that members of the 2012 mTBI cohort who had a history of deployment at the time of diagnosis were much more likely to receive treatment for an adjustment disorder, anxiety disorder, PTSD, and depression, compared with those who had never deployed ($p < 0.0001$). The most striking difference was that 15 percent of those who had deployed received treatment for PTSD, compared with 2.5 percent of those without a history of deployment ($p < 0.0001$). Alcohol abuse/dependence was not correlated with deployment history, however. In general, the higher rates of treatment for co-occurring behavioral health conditions among service members who have deployed is not surprising: Research has demonstrated a higher prevalence of these conditions as a consequence of combat deployment (Milliken, Auchterlonie, and Hoge, 2007; Seal et al., 2009; Thomas et al., 2010; Hoge, Auchterlonie, and Milliken, 2006).

Figure E.8
Treatment for Behavioral Health Conditions in the Six Months After mTBI Diagnosis, by Deployment History

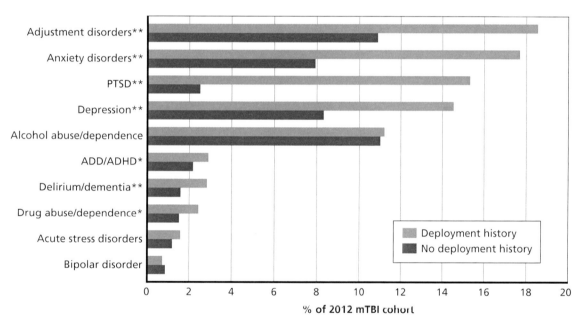

** Statistically significant difference at $p < 0.0001$.
 * Statistically significant difference at $p < 0.05$.

RAND RR844-E.8

We also considered differences in co-occurring conditions and symptoms by service and whether the individual had a history of deployment at the time of the mTBI diagnosis. Figure E.9 shows that there were differences by service for many of the conditions we assessed, though there were no differences by service in terms of receipt of treatment for skin sensation disturbances or smell and taste disturbances. As in the full cohort, treatment for non-headache pain conditions and headache were the most common conditions across the services. For most symptoms and conditions, Army personnel were more likely than other service members to have received treatment. For instance, 35 percent of Army personnel received treatment for sleep disorders, but this was significantly less common among other service members (approximately 10 percent of Navy and Air Force personnel and 20 percent of Marine Corps personnel received treatment for sleep problems). Army and Marine Corps personnel were three to four times more likely than Navy and Air Force personnel to have received treatment for memory loss in the six months following a new mTBI.

Figure E.9
Treatment for Symptoms and Conditions Commonly or Occasionally Co-Occurring with mTBI in the Six Months After Initial mTBI Diagnosis, by Service

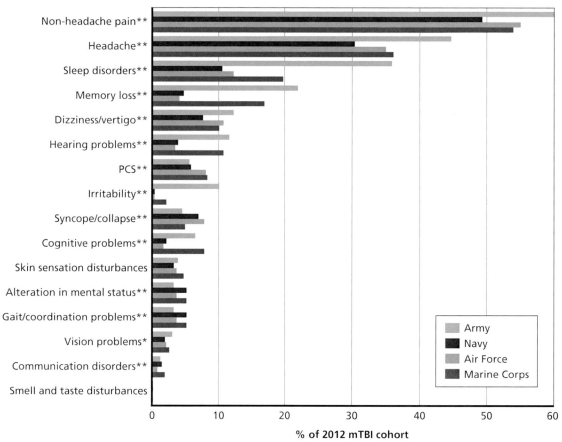

* Statistically significant difference at p < 0.03.
** Statistically significant difference at p < 0.0001.
RAND RR844-E.9

Figure E.10 shows that those with a history of deployment were generally more likely to experience the selected conditions and symptoms, with the exception of PCS and syncope, though differences in the prevalence of those conditions were very small. The largest differences across the two groups were in the rates of sleep disorders, memory loss, hearing problems, and irritability, with the group with a history of deployment much more likely than the non-deployers to have received treatment for these conditions (p < 0.0001).

Figure E.10
Treatment for Symptoms and Conditions Commonly or Occasionally Co-Occurring with mTBI in the Six Months After mTBI Diagnosis, by Deployment History

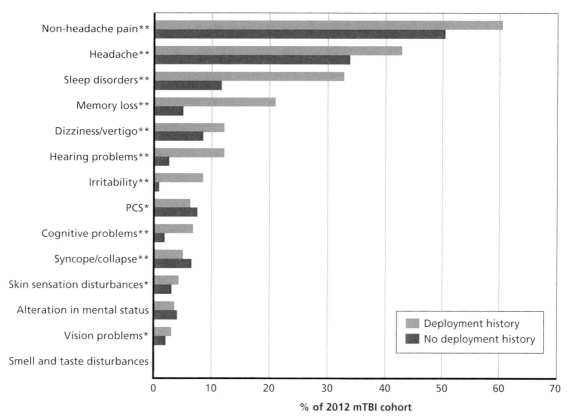

** Statistically significant difference at p < 0.0001.
 * Statistically significant difference at p < 0.01.

Table E.1 shows differences by service branch in the frequency of diagnostic assessments and evaluations received by service members with an mTBI in the six months following their diagnosis. All differences by service were statistically significant (p < 0.0001). Army personnel were less likely than personnel from the other services to receive a CT scan, for any reason, during this period. This may be explained, in part, by service differences in the location of care for the initial mTBI diagnosis. Compared with Army personnel, service members from other service branches were more likely to be diagnosed in civilian emergency departments, which may use CT scans more frequently than other settings or may order CT scans for conditions other than mTBI. The administrative data used in this analysis does not specify the purpose of the CT scan.

We also found that Army personnel with mTBI were most likely to receive a psychiatric diagnostic evaluation (36 percent), and Navy personnel were the least likely (14 percent). In fact, Army personnel were more likely to receive most of the assessments or evaluations in our analysis than were other service members.

Table E.1
Diagnostic Assessments and Evaluations Received in the Six Months After mTBI Diagnosis, by Service

Diagnostic Assessments	% of 2012 mTBI Cohort, by Service			
	Army	Navy	Air Force	Marine Corps
CT scan	21.2	46.1	48.7	42.6
Psychiatric diagnostic evaluation	35.8	14.4	23.5	25.1
Physical therapy evaluation	28.1	16.8	22.1	23.6
Neuropsychological assessment	14.1	4.5	9.0	10.5
Audiology examinations	10.9	10.1	4.1	15.2
Occupational therapy evaluation	12.7	5.4	3.9	10.0
Health and behavior assessment	12.1	6.5	0.8	9.9
Neurobehavioral status exam	13.1	1.0	1.5	2.0
Evaluation of speech, language, voice, communication, and/or auditory processing	6.2	2.8	1.2	11.2
Sleep study	6.6	2.2	1.9	3.8
Sensorimotor examination[a]	—	—	—	—
Vestibular testing	2.7	1.2	0.9	3.2

NOTE: All differences by service are statistically significant at p < 0.0001.

[a] Not reported because some cells had fewer than n = 20 service members.

Figure E.11 shows that service members with mTBI who had deployed were more likely to receive most of the diagnostic assessments during the six months after their mTBI diagnosis, compared with service members with mTBI who had not deployed (p < 0.0001).

Figure E.11
Diagnostic Assessments and Evaluations Received in the Six Months After mTBI Diagnosis, by Deployment History

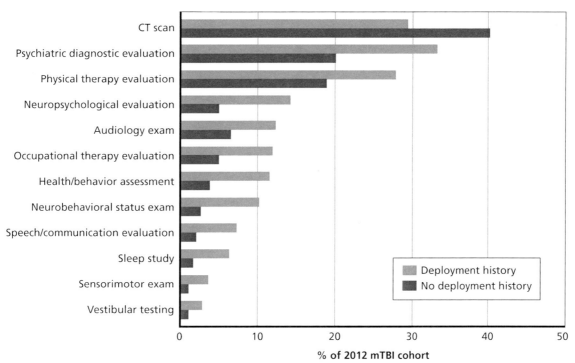

% of 2012 mTBI cohort

NOTES: Assessments and evaluations may be related to co-occurring conditions rather than mTBI. All differences statistically significant at p < 0.0001.

RAND *RR844-E.11*

When we examined differences in the receipt of various treatments by service branch (Table E.2), we found that Army and Marine Corps personnel were more likely than Navy and Air Force personnel to receive psychotherapy, CAM, and other therapies in the six months following their initial mTBI diagnosis (p < 0.001). While one explanation may be differences in the rates by service of co-occurring behavioral health and other conditions, these differences could also be due to variations in coding practice by service, availability of treatment resources, or other factors.

Table E.2
Therapies Received in the Six Months After mTBI Diagnosis, by Service

Therapy/Treatment Type	% of 2012 mTBI Cohort, by Service			
	Army	Navy	Air Force	Marine Corps
Psychotherapy (any)	38.9	14.4	18.5	25.9
Individual psychotherapy	36.7	13.7	17.2	24.7
Group psychotherapy	11.6	4.1	3.4	7.6
Family psychotherapy[a]	—	—	—	—
Physical therapy (therapeutic exercise, neuromuscular reeducation, physical therapy activities)	25.3	18.1	21.9	25.8
CAM (any)	11.6	7.4	8.4	11.2
Acupuncture	1.9	1.6	1.0	2.6
Chiropractic	5.0	3.7	3.3	4.8
Biofeedback[a]	—	—	—	—
Other CAM	5.3	2.8	5.0	3.3
Occupational therapy	8.9	5.3	3.6	10.4
Neuromuscular electrical stimulation	7.3	6.0	6.2	9.1
Speech therapy	7.6	3.0	1.3	12.6
Cognitive rehabilitation	7.6	1.2	0.7	6.4
Health and behavior intervention	4.3	3.7	1.2	5.0
CPAP/BiPAP	2.9	1.1	0.7	1.2
Sensory integration therapy[a]	—	—	—	—

NOTE: All differences by service are statistically significant at p < 0.001.

[a] Not reported because some cells had fewer than n = 20 service members.

Service members who had deployed were much more likely to receive various types of treatments in the six months following their mTBI diagnosis than were those who had never deployed (see Figure E.12). Thirty-five percent of those who had deployed received psychotherapy, compared with 19 percent of those who had not deployed (p < 0.0001), and 7 percent of those who had deployed received cognitive rehabilitation, compared with less than 2 percent of those who had not deployed (p < 0.0001).

Figure E.12
Therapies Received in the Six Months After Initial mTBI Diagnosis, by Deployment History

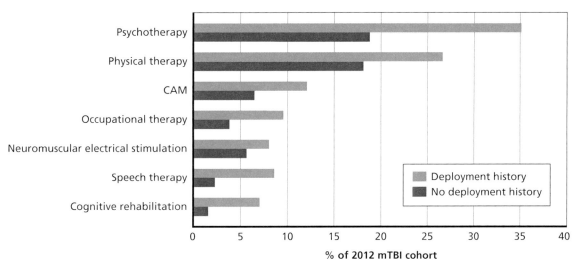

NOTES: Therapies may be related to co-occurring conditions rather than mTBI. All differences statistically significant at p < 0.0001.
RAND *RR844-E.12*

We also examined filled prescriptions by service and found some noticeable differences (Table E.3). For example, soldiers and marines with mTBI were more likely to fill a prescription for antidepressants and sleep aids compared to sailors or airmen.

We also observed differences in medication use between service members who had deployed and those who had not (see Figure E.13). There was no difference by deployment history in the use of analgesics and only a slight difference in the use of opioids (46 percent versus 44 percent, $p < 0.05$). Those who had deployed were twice as likely than those who had not to have filled a prescription for an antidepressant (29 percent versus 14 percent, $p < 0.0001$) or sleep aid (24 percent versus 11 percent, $p < 0.0001$). We found similar patterns for other medication types; in all cases, those who had deployed were more likely to have filled a prescription than were those who had not deployed. Many of these differences may be explained by differences in the prevalence of co-occurring diagnoses by deployment history, particularly behavioral health diagnoses.

Table E.3
Prescriptions Filled in the Six Months After mTBI Diagnosis, for Any Reason, by Service

Medication Type	% of 2012 mTBI Cohort, by Service			
	Army	Navy	Air Force	Marine Corps
Analgesics***	65.5	57.3	54.6	62.7
Opioids*	46.2	44.1	43.4	46.6
Antidepressants***	30.9	12.6	12.7	23.4
Sleep aids***	25.6	9.1	11.7	17.7
Muscle relaxants***	21.8	16.4	20.1	17.4
Anticonvulsants/mood stabilizers***	14.0	6.5	6.1	12.9
Headache medications***	13.8	5.0	3.5	7.3
Benzodiazepines***	12.8	7.7	9.5	9.7
Prazosin***	8.7	1.0	0.8	6.0
Antipsychotics***	5.4	1.5	1.0	4.4
Stimulants***	3.2	1.0	2.2	2.0
Alcohol/drug treatment**	1.3	0.6	0.6	0.9

NOTE: Analgesics include NSAIDs, acetaminophen, and other non-opioid analgesics.
*** Statistically significant difference at $p < 0.0001$.
** Statistically significant difference at $p < 0.001$.
* Statistically significant difference at $p < 0.05$.

Figure E.13
Prescriptions Filled in the Six Months After mTBI Diagnosis, for Any Reason, by Deployment History

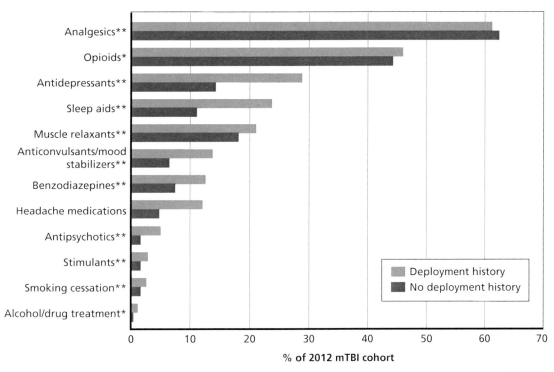

% of 2012 mTBI cohort

NOTES: Analgesics include NSAIDs, acetaminophen, and other non-opioid analgesics. Prescriptions may be related to co-occurring conditions rather than mTBI.

**Statistically significant difference at p < 0.0001.
*Statistically significant difference at p < 0.05.

RAND RR844-E.13

References

AFHSC—*See* Armed Forces Health Surveillance Center.

Agency for Healthcare Research and Quality, *Coordinating Care for Adults with Complex Care Needs in the Patient-Centered Medical Home: Challenges and Solutions*, Rockville, Md., January 2012. As of January 13, 2015:
http://pcmh.ahrq.gov/page/coordinating-care-adults-complex-care-needs-patient-centered-medical-home-challenges-and

AHRQ—*See* Agency for Healthcare Research and Quality.

Altmire, Jason, U.S. Representative from Pennsylvania, testimony on legislation affecting veterans before the Subcommittee on Health, Committee on Veterans' Affairs, U.S. House of Representatives, Washington, D.C., April 26, 2007.

Andelic, Nada, Solrun Sigurdardottir, Anne-Kristine Schanke, Leiv Sandvik, Unni Sveen, and Cecilie Roe, "Disability, Physical Health and Mental Health 1 Year After Traumatic Brain Injury," *Disability and Rehabilitation*, Vol. 32, No. 13, 2010, pp. 1122–1131.

Anstey, Kaarin J., Peter Butterworth, Anthony F. Jorm, Helen Christensen, Bryan Rodgers, and Timothy D. Windsor, "A Population Survey Found an Association Between Self-Reports of Traumatic Brain Injury and Increased Psychiatric Symptoms," *Journal of Clinical Epidemiology*, Vol. 57, No. 11, November 2004, pp. 1202–1209.

Armed Forces Health Surveillance Center, "Deriving Case Counts from Medical Encounter Data: Considerations When Interpreting Health Surveillance Reports," *Medical Surveillance Monthly Report*, Vol. 16, No. 12, December 2009, pp. 2–8.

———, "Section 13, Neurology," *AFHSC Case Definitions for Health Analysis and Data Reports*, Silver Spring, Md., 2012. As of January 13, 205:
http://www.afhsc.mil/documents/pubs/documents/CaseDefs/Web_13_NEUROLOGY_APR12.pdf

———, "Case Definition Development," *AFHSC Case Definitions for Health Analysis and Data Reports*, 2013. As of January 13, 2015:
http://www.afhsc.mil/documents/pubs/documents/CaseDefs/Web_Case_Definition_Development_JAN13.pdf

Bazarian, Jeffrey J., and Shireen Atabaki, "Predicting Postconcussion Syndrome After Minor Traumatic Brain Injury," *Academic Emergency Medicine*, Vol. 8, No. 8, August 2001, pp. 788–795.

Bazarian, Jeffrey J., Peter Veazie, Sohug Mookerjee, and E. Brooke Lerner, "Accuracy of Mild Traumatic Brain Injury Case Ascertainment Using ICD-9 Codes," *Academic Emergency Medicine*, Vol. 13, No. 1, January 2006, pp. 31–38.

Birman-Deych, Elena, Amy D. Waterman, Yan Yan, David S. Nilasena, Martha J. Radford, and Brian F. Gage, "Accuracy of ICD-9-CM Codes for Identifying Cardiovascular and Stroke Risk Factors," *Medical Care*, Vol. 43, No. 5, May 2005, pp. 480–485.

Bombardier, Charles H., Jesse R. Fann, Nancy R. Temkin, Peter C. Esselman, Jason Barber, and Sureyya S. Dikmen, "Rates of Major Depressive Disorder and Clinical Outcomes Following Traumatic Brain Injury," *Journal of the American Medical Association*, Vol. 303, No. 19, May 19, 2010, pp. 1938–1945.

Borg, Jörgen, Lena Holm, J. David Cassidy, Paul Peloso, Linda J. Carroll, Hans Von Holst, and Kaj Ericson, "Diagnostic Procedures in Mild Traumatic Brain Injury: Results of the WHO Collaborating Centre Task Force on Mild Traumatic Brain Injury," *Journal of Rehabilitation Medicine*, Vol. 36, Suppl. 43, 2004, pp. 61–75.

Borgaro, Susan R., George P. Prigatano, Christina Kwasnica, and Jennie L. Rexer, "Cognitive and Affective Sequelae in Complicated and Uncomplicated Mild Traumatic Brain Injury," *Brain Injury*, Vol. 17, No. 3, March 2003, pp. 189–198.

Brenner, Lisa A., Brian J. Ivins, Karen Schwab, Deborah Warden, Lonnie A. Nelson, Michael Jaffee, and Heidi Terrio, "Traumatic Brain Injury, Posttraumatic Stress Disorder, and Postconcussive Symptom Reporting among Troops Returning from Iraq," *Journal of Head Trauma Rehabilitation*, Vol. 25, No. 5, September–October 2010, pp. 307–312.

Brenner, Lisa A., Rodney D. Vanderploeg, and Heidi Terrio, "Assessment and Diagnosis of Mild Traumatic Brain Injury, Posttraumatic Stress Disorder, and Other Polytrauma Conditions: Burden of Adversity Hypothesis," *Rehabilitation Psychology*, Vol. 54, No. 3, August 2009, pp. 239–246.

Bryant, Richard A., "Posttraumatic Stress Disorder and Mild Brain Injury: Controversies, Causes and Consequences," *Journal of Clinical and Experimental Neuropsychology*, Vol. 23, No. 6, 2010, pp. 718–728.

Cameron, Kenneth L., Stephen W. Marshall, Rodney X. Sturdivant, and Andrew E. Lincoln, "Trends in the Incidence of Physician-Diagnosed Mild Traumatic Brain Injury Among Active Duty U.S. Military Personnel Between 1997 and 2007," *Journal of Neurotrauma*, Vol. 29, No. 7, May 1, 2012, pp. 1313–1321.

Carlson, Kathleen F., Shannon M. Kehle, Laura A. Meis, Nancy Greer, Roderick Macdonald, Indulis Rutks, Nina A. Sayer, Steven K. Dobscha, and Timothy J. Wilt, "Prevalence, Assessment, and Treatment of Mild Traumatic Brain Injury and Posttraumatic Stress Disorder: A Systematic Review of the Evidence," *Journal of Head Trauma Rehabilitation*, Vol. 26, No. 2, March–April 2011, pp. 103–115.

Carroll, Linda J., J. David Cassidy, Carol Cancelliere, Pierre Côté, Cesar A. Hincapié, Vicki L. Kristman, Lena W. Holm, Jörgen Borg, Catharina Nygren-de Boussard, and Jan Hartvigsen, "Systematic Review of the Prognosis After Mild Traumatic Brain Injury in Adults: Cognitive, Psychiatric, and Mortality Outcomes: Results of the International Collaboration on Mild Traumatic Brain Injury Prognosis," *Archives of Physical Medicine and Rehabilitation*, Vol. 95, No. 3, Suppl., March 2014, pp. S152–S173.

Chen, Amy Y., and Angela Colantonio, "Defining Neurotrauma in Administrative Data Using the International Classification of Diseases Tenth Revision," *Emerging Themes in Epidemiology*, Vol. 8, No. 4, 2011.

Clark, John, "Casualty of War," *Newsweek*, March 16, 2006.

Coronado, Victor G., Likang Xu, Sridhar V. Basavaraju, Lisa C. McGuire, Marlena M. Wald, Mark D. Faul, Bernardo R. Guzman, and John D. Hemphill, *Surveillance for Traumatic Brain Injury-Related Deaths: United States, 1997–2007*, Atlanta, Ga.: Centers for Disease Control and Prevention, 2011.

Consumer Assessment of Healthcare Providers and Systems, Agency for Healthcare Research and Quality, homepage, undated. As of January 13, 2015:
https://cahps.ahrq.gov

Dean, Philip J., Darragh O'Neill, and Annette Sterr, "Post-Concussion Syndrome: Prevalence after Mild Traumatic Brain Injury in Comparison with a Sample Without Head Injury," *Brain Injury*, Vol. 26, No. 1, January 2012, pp. 14–26.

DCoE—*See* Defense Centers of Excellence for Psychological Health and Traumatic Brain Injury.

Defense and Veterans Brain Injury Center, "Concussion/Mild Traumatic Brain Injury Rehabilitation: Headache and Neck Pain," fact sheet, 2009.

———, "Personal Communication," April 2013.

———, "DoD Worldwide Numbers for TBI," web page, 2014a. As of September 30, 2014:
http://dvbic.dcoe.mil/dod-worldwide-numbers-tbi

———, *DoD Worldwide Numbers for TBI: 2012 Annual Report*, Silver Spring, Md., 2014b. As of January 13, 2015:
http://dvbic.dcoe.mil/sites/default/files/Worldwide-Totals-2012.pdf

———, "Progressive Return to Activity Following Acute Concussion/Mild Traumatic Brain Injury," 2014c. As of January 13, 2015:
http://dvbic.dcoe.mil/resources/progressive-return-to-activity

Defense and Veterans Brain Injury Center Working Group on Acute Management of Mild Traumatic Brain Injury in Military Operational Settings, *Clinical Practice Guideline and Recommendations*, December 22, 2006. As of January 13, 2015:
http://www.pdhealth.mil/downloads/clinical_practice_guideline_recommendations.pdf

Defense Centers of Excellence for Psychological Health and Traumatic Brain Injury, *Assessment and Management of Dizziness Associated with Mild TBI*, September 2012. As of January 13, 2015:
http://www.dcoe.mil/content/Navigation/Documents/Dizziness_Associated_with_Mild_TBI_Clinical_Recommendation.pdf

Defense Centers of Excellence for Psychological Health and Traumatic Brain Injury and Defense and Veterans Brain Injury Center, *Mild Traumatic Brain Injury Pocket Guide (CONUS)*, 2010. As of January 13, 2015:
http://www.dcoe.mil/Content/Navigation/Documents/Mild%20Traumatic%20Brain%20Injury%20Pocket%20Guide.pdf

DoD—*See* U.S. Department of Defense.

DVBIC—*See* Defense and Veterans Brain Injury Center.

Eibner, Christine, Jeanne S. Ringel, Beau Kilmer, Rosalie Liccardo Pacula, and Claudia Diaz, "The Cost of Post-Deployment Mental Health and Cognitive Conditions," in Terri Tanielian and Lisa H. Jaycox, eds., *Invisible Wounds of War*, Santa Monica, Calif.: RAND Corporation, MG-720-CCF, 2008, pp. 169–234. As of January 13, 2015:
http://www.rand.org/pubs/monographs/MG720.html

Farace, Elana, and Wayne M. Alves, "Do Women Fare Worse? A Metaanalysis of Gender Differences in Outcome After Traumatic Brain Injury," *Journal of Neurosurgery*, Vol. 93, No. 4, October 2000, pp. 395–345.

Faul, Mark, Likang Xu, Marlena M. Wald, and Victor G. Coronado, *Traumatic Brain Injury in the United States: Emergency Department Visits, Hospitalizations and Deaths 2002–2006*, Atlanta, Ga.: Centers for Disease Control and Prevention, National Center for Injury Prevention and Control, March 2010. As of January 13, 2015:
http://www.cdc.gov/traumaticbraininjury/pdf/blue_book.pdf

Fenton, George, Roy McClelland, Anne Montgomery, Geraldine MacFlynn, and William Rutherford, "The Postconcussional Syndrome: Social Antecedents and Psychological Sequelae," *British Journal of Psychiatry*, Vol. 162, April 1993, pp. 493–497.

Guinto, Gerardo, and Yoshiaki Guinto-Nishimura, "Postconcussion Syndrome: A Complex and Underdiagnosed Clinical Entity," *World Neurosurgery*, Vol. 82, No. 5, November 2014, pp. 627–628.

Guskiewicz, Kevin M., Stephen W. Marshall, Julian Bailes, Michael McCrea, Robert C. Cantu, Christopher Randolph, and Barry D. Jordan, "Association Between Recurrent Concussion and Late-Life Cognitive Impairment in Retired Professional Football Players," *Neurosurgery*, Vol. 57, No. 4, October 2005, pp. 719–726.

Hartlage, Lawrence C., Denise Durant-Wilson, and Peter C. Patch, "Persistent Neurobehavioral Problems Following Mild Traumatic Brain Injury," *Archives of Clinical Neuropsychology*, Vol. 16, No. 6, August 2001, pp. 561–570.

Helmick, Kathy, Laura Baugh, Tracy Lattimore, and Sarah Goldman, "Traumatic Brain Injury: Next Steps, Research Needed, and Priority Focus Areas," *Military Medicine*, Vol. 177, No. 8, Suppl., August 2012, pp. 86–92.

Hoge, Charles W., Jennifer L. Auchterlonie, and Charles S. Milliken, "Mental Health Problems, Use of Mental Health Services, and Attrition from Military Service After Returning from Deployment to Iraq or Afghanistan," *Journal of the American Medical Association*, Vol. 295, No. 9, March 1, 2006, pp. 1023–1032.

Hoge, Charles W., Herb M. Goldberg, and Carl A. Castro, "Care of War Veterans with Mild Traumatic Brain Injury—Flawed Perspectives," *New England Journal of Medicine*, Vol. 360, April 16, 2009, pp. 1588–1591.

Hoge, Charles W., Dennis McGurk, Jeffrey L. Thomas, Anthony L. Cox, Charles C. Engel, and Carl A. Castro, "Mild Traumatic Brain Injury in US Soldiers Returning from Iraq," *New England Journal of Medicine*, Vol. 358, January 31, 2008, pp. 453–463.

Hunt, John P., Christopher C. Baker, Samir M. Fakhry, Robert R. Rutledge, David Ransohoff, and Anthony A. Meyer, "Accuracy of Administrative Data in Trauma," *Surgery*, Vol. 126, No. 2, August 1999, pp. 191–197.

Hyatt, Kyong, Linda L. Davis, and Julie Barroso, "Chasing the Care: Soldiers Experience Following Combat-Related Mild Traumatic Brain Injury," *Military Medicine*, Vol. 179, No. 8, August 2014, pp. 849–855.

"Incident Diagnoses of Common Symptoms ('Sequelae') Following Traumatic Brain Injury, Active Component, U.S. Armed Forces, 2000–2012," *Medical Surveillance Monthly Report*, Vol. 20, No. 6, June 2013, pp. 9–13.

Kristman, Vicki L., Jörgen Borg, Alison K. Godbolt, L. Rachid Salmi, Carol Cancelliere, Linda J. Carroll, Lena W. Holm, Catharina Nygren-de Boussard, Jan Hartvigsen, Uko Abara, James Donovan, and J. David Cassidy, "Methodological Issues and Research Recommendations for Prognosis After Mild Traumatic Brain Injury: Results of the International Collaboration on Mild Traumatic Brain Injury Prognosis," *Archives of Physical Medicine and Rehabilitation*, Vol. 95, No. 3, Suppl., March 2014, pp. S265–S277.

Laborde, Andrea, "NIH Consensus Development Panel on Rehabilitation of Persons with Traumatic Brain Injury," *Journal of Head Trauma Rehabilitation*, Vol. 15, No. 1, February 2000, pp. 761–763.

Lagarde, Emmanuel, Louis-Rachid Salmi, Lena W. Holm, Benjamin Contrand, François Masson, Régis Ribéreau-Gayon, Magali Laborey, and J. David Cassidy, "Association of Symptoms Following Mild Traumatic Brain Injury with Posttraumatic Stress Disorder vs Postconcussion Syndrome," *JAMA Psychiatry*, Vol. 71, No. 9, September 1, 2014, pp. 1032–1040.

Lew, Henry L., John D. Otis, Carlos Tun, Robert D. Kerns, Michael E. Clark, and David X. Cifu, "Prevalence of Chronic Pain, Posttraumatic Stress Disorder, and Persistent Postconcussive Symptoms in OIF/OEF Veterans: Polytrauma Clinical Triad," *Journal of Rehabilitation Research and Development*, Vol. 46, No. 6, July 2009, pp. 697–702.

Lew, Henry L., Terri K. Pogoda, Errol Baker, Kelly L. Stolzmann, Mark Meterko, David X. Cifu, Jomana Amara, and Ann M. Hendricks, "Prevalence of Dual Sensory Impairment and Its Association with Traumatic Brain Injury and Blast Exposure in OEF/OIF Veterans," *Journal of Head Trauma Rehabilitation*, Vol. 26, No. 6, November–December 2011, pp. 489–496.

Lew, Henry L., John H. Poole, Rodney D. Vanderploeg, Gregory L. Goodrich, Sharon Dekelboum, Sylvia B. Guillory, Barbara Sigford, and David X. Cifu, "Program Development and Defining Characteristics of Returning Military in a Va Polytrauma Network Site," *Journal of Rehabilitation Research and Development*, Vol. 44, No. 7, 2007, pp. 1027–1034.

Lloyd, Susan S., and J. Peter Rissing, "Physician and Coding Errors in Patient Records," *Journal of the American Medical Association*, Vol. 254, No. 10, September 13, 1985, pp. 1330–1336.

Logan, Bret W., Sarah Goldman, Mark Zola, and Angela Mackey, "Concussive Brain Injury in the Military: September 2001 to the Present," *Behavioral Sciences and the Law*, Vol. 31, No. 6, November–December 2013, pp. 803–813.

Lundin, A., C. de Boussard, G. Edman, and J. Borg, "Symptoms and Disability Until 3 Months After Mild TBI," *Brain Injury*, Vol. 20, No. 8, 2006, pp. 799–806.

MacGregor, Andrew J., Richard A. Shaffer, Amber L. Dougherty, Michael R. Galarneau, Rema Raman, Dewleen G. Baker, Suzanne P. Lindsay, Beatrice A. Golomb, and Karen S. Corson, "Prevalence and Psychological Correlates of Traumatic Brain Injury in Operation Iraqi Freedom," *Journal of Head Trauma Rehabilitation*, Vol. 25, No. 1, January–February 2010, pp. 1–8.

MacIntyre, C. Raina, Michael J. Ackland, and Eugene J. Chandraraj, "Accuracy of Injury Coding in Victorian Hospital Morbidity Data," *Australian and New Zealand Journal of Public Health*, Vol. 21, No. 7, December 1997, pp. 779–783.

Manley, Geoffrey T., and Andrew I. R. Maas, "Traumatic Brain Injury: An International Knowledge-Based Approach," *Journal of the American Medical Association*, Vol. 310, No. 5, August 7, 2013, pp. 473–474.

Marr, Angela L., and Victor G. Coronado, *Central Nervous System Injury Surveillance Data Submission Standards—2002*, Atlanta, Ga.: Centers for Disease Control and Prevention, National Center for Injury Prevention and Control, 2004.

Martin, Laurie T., Coreen Farris, Andrew M. Parker, and Caroline Epley, *The Defense and Veterans Brain Injury Center Care Coordination Program: Assessment of Program Structure, Activities, and Implementation*, Santa Monica, Calif.: RAND Corporation, RR-126-OSD, 2013. As of January 13, 2015: http://www.rand.org/pubs/research_reports/RR126.html

McCrea, Michael, Kevin M. Guskiewicz, Stephen W. Marshall, William Barr, Christopher Randolph, Robert C. Cantu, James A. Onate, Jingzhen Yang, and James P. Kelly, "Acute Effects and Recovery Time Following Concussion in Collegiate Football Players: The NCAA Concussion Study," *Journal of the American Medical Association*, Vol. 290, No. 19, November 19, 2003, pp. 2556–2563.

McCrea, Michael, Grant L. Iverson, Thomas W. McAllister, Thomas A. Hammeke, Matthew R. Powell, William B. Barr, and James P. Kelly, "An Integrated Review of Recovery After Mild Traumatic Brain Injury (MTBI): Implications for Clinical Management," *Clinical Neuropsychologist*, Vol. 23, 2009, pp. 1368–1390.

Miller, Shannon C., Suzanne H. Baktash, Timothy S. Webb, Casserly R. Whitehead, Charles Maynard, Timothy S. Wells, Clifford N. Otte, and Russel K. Gore, "Risk for Addiction-Related Disorders Following Mild Traumatic Brain Injury in a Large Cohort of Active-Duty U.S. Airmen," *American Journal of Psychiatry*, Vol. 170, No. 4, April 2013, pp. 383–390.

Milliken, Charles S., Jennifer L. Auchterlonie, and Charles W. Hoge, "Longitudinal Assessment of Mental Health Problems Among Active and Reserve Component Soldiers Returning from the Iraq War," *Journal of the American Medical Association*, Vol. 298, No. 18, November 14, 2007, pp. 2141–2148.

National Center for Health Statistics, *International Classification of Diseases, Ninth Revision, Clinical Modification (ICD-9-CM)*, Atlanta, Ga., June 18, 2013. As of January 13, 2015: http://www.cdc.gov/nchs/icd/icd9cm.htm

National Center for Injury Prevention and Control, Centers for Disease Control and Prevention, *Report to Congress on Mild Traumatic Brain Injury in the United States: Steps to Prevent a Serious Public Health Problem*, Atlanta, Ga., 2003.

National Institute of Neurological Disorders and Stroke, "NINDS Traumatic Brain Injury Information Page," last updated July 22, 2014. As of January 13, 2015: http://www.ninds.nih.gov/disorders/tbi/tbi.htm

Nicholson, Keith, "Pain, Cognition and Traumatic Brain Injury," *NeuroRehabilitation*, Vol. 14, No. 2, 2000, pp. 95–103.

Novack, Thomas A., Amy L. Alderson, Beverly A. Bush, Jay M. Meythaler, and Kay Canupp, "Cognitive and Functional Recovery at 6 and 12 Months Post-TBI," *Brain Injury*, Vol. 14, No. 11, November 2000, pp. 987–996.

Office of the Surgeon General, *TBI Talking Points 2013*, Washington, D.C., 2013.

Orman, Jean A. Langlois, Anbersaw W. Selassie, Christopher L. Perdue, David J. Thurman, and Jess F. Kraus, "Surveillance of Traumatic Brain Injury," in Li Guohua and Susan P. Baker, eds., *Injury Research: Theories, Methods, and Approaches*, New York: Springer, 2012, pp. 61–86.

Packard, Russell C., Richard Weaver, and Lesley P. Ham, "Cognitive Symptoms in Patients with Posttraumatic Headache," *Headache*, Vol. 33, No. 7, July–August 1993, pp. 365–368.

Peabody, John W., Jeff Luck, Sharad Jain, Dan Bertenthal, and Peter Glassman, "Assessing the Accuracy of Administrative Data in Health Information Systems," *Medical Care*, Vol. 42, No. 11, November 2004, pp. 1066–1072.

Perlis, Michael L., Lydia Artiola, and Donna E. Giles, "Sleep Complaints in Chronic Postconcussion Syndrome," *Perceptual and Motor Skills*, Vol. 84, No. 2, April 1997, pp. 595–599.

Ponsford, Jennie, Catherine Willmott, Andrew Rothwell, Peter Cameron, A. M. Kelly, Robyn Nelms, Carolyn Curran, and Kim Ng, "Factors Influencing Outcome Following Mild Traumatic Brain Injury in Adults," *Journal of the International Neuropsychological Society*, Vol. 6, No. 5, July 2000, pp. 568–579.

Powell, Janet M., Joseph V. Ferraro, Sureyya S. Dikmen, Nancy R. Temkin, and Kathleen R. Bell, "Accuracy of Mild Traumatic Brain Injury Diagnosis," *Archives of Physical Medicine and Rehabilitation*, Vol. 89, No. 8, August 2008, pp. 1550–1555.

Reddy, Cara Camiolo, "Postconcussion Syndrome: A Physiatrist's Approach," *PM&R*, Vol. 3, No. 10, Suppl. 2, October 2011, pp. S396–S405.

Rockhill, Carol Mary, Kenneth Jaffe, Chuan Zhou, Ming-Yu Fan, Wayne Katon, and Jesse R. Fann, "Health Care Costs Associated with Traumatic Brain Injury and Psychiatric Illness in Adults," *Journal of Neurotrauma*, Vol. 29, No. 6, 2012, pp. 1038–1046.

Roozenbeek, Bob, Andrew I. Maas, and David K. Menon, "Changing Patterns in the Epidemiology of Traumatic Brain Injury," *Nature Reviews Neurology*, Vol. 9, No. 4, 2013, pp. 231–236.

Ruff, Ronald, "Two Decades of Advances in Understanding of Mild Traumatic Brain Injury," *Journal of Head Trauma Rehabilitation*, Vol. 20, No. 1, January–February 2005, pp. 5–18.

Ryan, Laurie M., and Deborah L. Warden, "Post Concussion Syndrome," *International Review of Psychiatry*, Vol. 15, No. 4, November 2003, pp. 310–316.

Schatz, Philip, Rosemarie Scolaro Moser, Tracey Covassin, and Robin Karpf, "Early Indicators of Enduring Symptoms in High School Athletes with Multiple Previous Concussions," *Neurosurgery*, Vol. 68, No. 6, 2011, pp. 1562–1567.

Schell, Terry L., and Grant N. Marshall, "Survey of Individuals Previously Deployed for OEF/OIF," in Terri Tanielian and Lisa H. Jaycox, eds., *Invisible Wounds of War: Psychological and Cognitive Injuries, Their Consequences, and Services to Assist Recovery*, Santa Monica, Calif.: RAND Corporation, MG-720-CCF, 2008, pp. 87–113. As of January 13, 2015:
http://www.rand.org/pubs/monographs/MG720.html

Schneiderman, Aaron I., Elisa R. Braver, and Han K. Kang, "Understanding Sequelae of Injury Mechanisms and Mild Traumatic Brain Injury Incurred During the Conflicts in Iraq and Afghanistan: Persistent Postconcussive Symptoms and Posttraumatic Stress Disorder," *American Journal of Epidemiology*, Vol. 167, No. 12, June 15, 2008, pp. 1446–1452.

Seal, Karen H., Thomas J. Metzler, Kristian S. Gima, Daniel Bertenthal, Shira Maguen, and Charles R. Marmar, "Trends and Risk Factors for Mental Health Diagnoses Among Iraq and Afghanistan Veterans Using Department of Veterans Affairs Health Care, 2002–2008," *American Journal of Public Health*, Vol. 99, No. 9, September 2009, pp. 1651–1658.

Shore, Andrew D., Melissa L. McCarthy, Tracey Serpi, and Melanie Gertner, "Validity of Administrative Data for Characterizing Traumatic Brain Injury-Related Hospitalizations," *Brain Injury*, Vol. 19, No. 8, August 2005, pp. 613–621.

Spira, James L., Corinna E. Lathan, Joseph Bleiberg, and Jack W. Tsao, "The Impact of Multiple Concussions on Emotional Distress, Postconcussive Symptoms, and Neurocognitive Functioning, in Active Duty United States Marines Independent of Combat Exposure or Emotional Distress," *Journal of Neurotrauma*, Vol. 31, No. 22, November 15, 2014, pp. 1823–1834.

Stein, Murray B., and Thomas W. McAllister, "Exploring the Convergence of Posttraumatic Stress Disorder and Mild Traumatic Brain Injury," *American Journal of Psychiatry*, Vol. 166, No. 7, July 2009, pp. 768–776.

Taylor, Brent C., Emily M. Hagel, Kathleen F. Carlson, David X. Cifu, Andrea Cutting, Douglas E. Bidelspach, and Nina A. Sayer, "Prevalence and Costs of Co-Occurring Traumatic Brain Injury with and Without Psychiatric Disturbance and Pain Among Afghanistan and Iraq War Veteran V.A. Users," *Medical Care*, Vol. 50, No. 4, 2012, pp. 342–346.

Thomas, Jeffrey L., Joshua E. Wilk, Lyndon A. Riviere, Dennis McGurk, Carl A. Castro, and Charles W. Hoge, "Prevalence of Mental Health Problems and Functional Impairment Among Active Component and National Guard Soldiers 3 and 12 Months Following Combat in Iraq," *Archives of General Psychiatry*, Vol. 67, No. 6, 2010, pp. 614–623.

Thornhill, Sharon, Graham M. Teasdale, Gordon D. Murray, James McEwen, Christopher W. Roy, and Kay I. Penny, "Disability in Young People and Adults One Year After Head Injury: Prospective Cohort Study," *British Medical Journal*, Vol. 320, No. 7250, June 17, 2000, pp. 1631–1635.

TRICARE, "Unified Biostatistical Utility (UBU): Coding Guidelines," web page, undated. As of January 13, 2015:
http://www.tricare.mil/ocfo/bea/ubu/coding_guidelines.cfm

U.S. Department of Defense, "Department of Defense Coding Guidance for Traumatic Brain Injury Fact Sheet," version 5.0, September 2010. As of January 13, 2015:
http://www.dcoe.mil/content/navigation/documents/Department%20of%20Defense%20Coding%20 Guidance%20for%20Traumatic%20Brain%20Injury%20Fact%20Sheet.pdf

———, *2012 Demographics: Profile of the Military Community*, Washington, D.C., 2013. As of January 13, 2015:
http://www.militaryonesource.mil/12038/MOS/Reports/2012_Demographics_Report.pdf

———, U.S. casualty status tables, web page, data as of December 31, 2014. No longer available online.

U.S. Department of Health and Human Services, "Administrative Simplification: Change to the Compliance Date for the International Classification of Diseases, 10th Revision (ICD-10-CM and ICD-10-PCS) Medical Data Code Sets," *Federal Register*, August 4, 2014. As of January 13, 2015:
https://www.federalregister.gov/articles/2014/08/04/2014-18347/ administrative-simplification-change-to-the-compliance-date-for-the-international-classification-of

U.S. Department of Veterans Affairs, *Independent Course on Traumatic Brain Injury*, April 2010. As of January 13, 2015:
http://www.publichealth.va.gov/docs/vhi/traumatic-brain-injury-vhi.pdf

U.S. Department of Veterans Affairs and U.S. Department of Defense, *Clinical Practice Guideline: Management of Concussion/Mild Traumatic Brain Injury*, version 1.0, Washington, D.C., April 2009. As of January 13, 2015:
http://www.healthquality.va.gov/guidelines/Rehab/mtbi/concussion_mtbi_full_1_0.pdf

VA—*See* U.S. Department of Veterans Affairs.

Vaishnavi, Sandeep, Vani Rao, and Jesse R. Fann, "Neuropsychiatric Problems After Traumatic Brain Injury: Unraveling the Silent Epidemic," *Psychosomatics*, Vol. 50, No. 3, May–June 2009, pp. 198–205.

Vanderploeg, Rodney D., Heather G. Belanger, and Glenn Curtiss, "Mild Traumatic Brain Injury and Posttraumatic Stress Disorder and Their Associations with Health Symptoms," *Archives of Physical Medicine and Rehabilitation*, Vol. 90, No. 7, July 2009, pp. 1084–1093.

Warden, Deborah, "Military TBI During the Iraq and Afghanistan Wars," *Journal of Head Trauma Rehabilitation*, Vol. 21, No. 5, September–October, 2006, pp. 398–402.

Wilde, Elisabeth A., Gale G. Whiteneck, Jennifer Bogner, Tamara Bushnik, David X. Cifu, Sureyya Dikmen, Louis French, Joseph T. Giacino, Tessa Harr, James F. Malec, Scott S. Tulsky, Rodney D. Vanderploeg, and Nicole von Steinbuechel, "Recommendations for the Use of Common Outcome Measures in Traumatic Brain Injury Research," *Archives of Physical Medicine and Rehabilitation*, Vol. 91, No. 11, November 2010, pp. 1650–1660.

Wilk, Joshua E., Richard K. Herrell, Gary H. Wynn, Lyndon A. Riviere, and Charles W. Hoge, "Mild Traumatic Brain Injury (Concussion), Posttraumatic Stress Disorder, and Depression in U.S. Soldiers Involved in Combat Deployments: Association with Postdeployment Symptoms," *Psychosomatic Medicine*, Vol. 74, No. 3, April 2012, pp. 249–257.

Wilson, Clay, *Improvised Explosive Devices (IEDs) in Iraq and Afghanistan: Effects and Countermeasures*, Washington, D.C.: Congressional Research Service, September 25, 2006.

Wojcik, Barbara E., Catherine R. Stein, Karen Bagg, Rebecca J. Humphrey, and Jason Orosco, "Traumatic Brain Injury Hospitalizations of U.S. Army Soldiers Deployed to Afghanistan and Iraq," *American Journal of Preventive Medicine*, Vol. 38, No. 1, 2010, pp. S108–S116.

Wynn, Alex, Matthew Wise, Mary Jo Wright, Aml Rafaat, Y. Z. Wang, Glen Steeb, Norman McSwain, Kennan J. Beuchter, and John P. Hunt, "Accuracy of Administrative and Trauma Registry Databases," *Journal of Trauma*, Vol. 51, No. 3, September 2001, pp. 464–468.